Peripheral
Nerve Blockade

For Churchill Livingstone

Commissioning Editor: Gavin Smith
Copy Editor: Penelope Lyons
Project Controller: Sarah Lowe
Text Design: Sarah Cape
Cover Design: Andrew Jones

Sciatic 20ml of
Levobupiv 0.375%

Peripheral Nerve Blockade

C. A. Pinnock MB BS FRCA

H. B. J. Fischer MB CHB FRCA

R. P. Jones MB CHB DA(UK)

Department of Anaesthesia
Alexandra Hospital
Woodrow Drive
Redditch
Worcestershire
UK

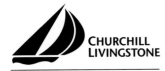

CHURCHILL
LIVINGSTONE

EDINBURGH LONDON NEW YORK PHILADELPHIA SAN FRANCISCO SYDNEY AND TORONTO 1998

CHURCHILL LIVINGSTONE
An imprint of Harcourt Brace and Company Limited

First published 1996
  Reprinted 1998

ISBN 0 443 05064 3

While great care has been taken to ensure the accuracy of
the book's content when it went to press, neither the
authors nor the publishers can be responsible for the
accuracy and completeness of the information. If there is
any doubt, the manufacturer's current literature or other
suitable reference should be consulted.

British Library Cataloguing in Publication Data
A catalogue record for this book is available from the
British Library

Library of Congress Cataloging in Publication Data
A catalog record for this book is available from the
Library of Congress

The
publisher's
policy is to use
**paper manufactured
from sustainable forests**

Produced by Addison Wesley Longman Singapore Pte Ltd
Printed in Singapore

Foreword

It was a pleasure to be asked to write a foreword for this book as it gave me a chance to learn from the manuscript and update my knowledge even before the book was published! I have no doubt that it is a most welcome addition to current books in the field of regional anaesthesia, a form of anaesthesia that is still very neglected in many geographical areas, but which has an important role in the provision of safe and effective pain relief for a wide variety of surgical procedures. The concept of the patient being awake during an operation is becoming far more widely accepted by anaesthetists, surgeons and particularly patients who are all learning of the considerable advantages to be gained. The judicious addition of sedation or even light general anaesthesia extends still further the number of patients who might benefit from the techniques described.

The development of newer and improved local anaesthetic agents, the use of adjuvants such as vasoconstrictors and perhaps opioids and α-receptor agonists, as well as the development of continuous techniques are all extending the potential of regional blocks. The techniques lend themselves very well to the increasing use and demand for day surgery, providing not only excellent anaesthesia with afferent blockade, but also optimal and often prolonged post-operative analgesia and sympathetic blockade.

It is difficult to think of any other group of anaesthetists who have more experience of this type of anaesthesia, or who are better qualified to transmit their vast experience of the techniques described. The authors have devoted much time to the teaching of many trainees who have passed through their hands, and have always welcomed others who may have had difficulty acquiring the relevant experience in their own hospitals and have sought the authors' help.

Methods are described that are most useful and widely applicable. The pages are full of information and guidance to ensure the correct choice of technique and then the accurate placement of the solution so that the highest success rate can be achieved with the minimum of complications, the goal of all anaesthetic techniques. The book will be a valuable and lasting source of information for anaesthetists at all levels, and I trust that examination candidates will assimilate its contents before their examiners do!

Dr Anthony Rubin
Consultant Anaesthetist
Charing Cross Hospital
London

Preface

The origins of this book lie in the practical experience we have gained in performing and teaching regional anaesthesia. We have committed our philosophy of regional anaesthesia to print in the hope that it might encourage others to offer patients the benefits of pain-free surgery. The last decade has produced a wealth of scientific and clinical evidence that demonstrates the benefits that can be attributed to the provision of good quality post-operative pain relief. The surge of interest in the management of acute pain is a testament to that goal. Local anaesthetic drugs are currently the only means of preventing nocioceptive stimuli from reaching the higher centres of pain perception and thus providing real opportunity of divorcing surgery from pain.

In the rush to promote the various benefits of central neural blockade, patient-controlled analgesia, and other systemic treatment regimens, the role of peripheral nerve blockade has been somewhat overlooked, so many patients undergoing surgery are denied the advantages that peripheral nerve blockade can offer in a wide variety of operations.

During this same decade of major advances in acute pain management, a generation of trainee anaesthetists has passed through the Department of Anaesthesia at the Alexandra Hospital, Redditch, itself only an embryo in 1986. We owe those trainees a debt of thanks for the impetus they provided that resulted in the writing of this volume. Whilst in post and on returning to visit us, they have posed the question 'Why don't you write a book?' as we slowly realised that our aims of providing and teaching simple, successful regional anaesthesia had stimulated an interest in the subject that went beyond our aims of departmental training.

We believe that this book differs from existing works by concentrating on the essentially practical nature of the subject. Our efforts have been directed towards providing a source of hands-on expertise which is based on our everyday working practice. The book is designed to be accessible to experienced practitioners (who will no doubt consult Section 3 directly to refresh their memory about a particular block) and to novices who will be able to divine from Section 2 which nerve blocks are indicated for the surgeon's intended operative site and thence move on to the appropriate techniques.

It is beyond the scope of this volume to enter into the theoretical aspects of pharmacology and neurophysiology that are extensively referenced in Section 4 for those readers needing further detail. The purpose of this book is to encourage those who wish to practise successful regional anaesthesia by offering clear advice and helpful tips. However, there is no substitute for the teaching of a skilled mentor.

We are grateful to our colleagues for their forbearance during the writing of this book, which is essentially the result of departmental collaboration. It is a tribute to them that regional anaesthesia is so widely practised within our hospital, an important factor in making this book easier to compile than it might otherwise have been.

Finally, we owe a debt of thanks to the department of EMIS at St. Bartholomew's Hospital for the excellence of their illustrations and to Braun UK for financially sponsoring the artwork.

CAP
HBJF
RPJ   Redditch 1996

Acknowledgements

EMIS, Education and Medical Illustration Services, St Bartholomew's Hospital, West Smithfield, London EC1A 7BE provided the artwork. The diagrams were drawn by Gareth Wild.

BRAUN, B Braun Medical Ltd, Braun House, Aylesbury Vale Industrial Park, Aylesbury, Bucks HP20 1DQ sponsored the artwork.

B–D, Becton Dickinson UK Ltd, Between Towns Road, Cowley, Oxford, OX4 3LY provided details of needle tips.

PHARMAPLAS (Steriseal Division), Thornhill Road, Redditch, Worcs. B98 9NL provided information on needle design.

Contents

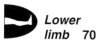
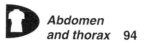
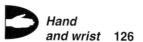
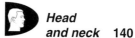
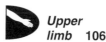

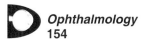 **Ophthalmology**
154

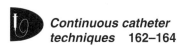 **Continuous catheter techniques   162–164**

SECTION 4
Reference   165

How to use this book

We have designed the book to be equally accessible to novice practitioners with an interest in regional anaesthesia and more senior personnel requiring refreshment of their skills. It is recommended strongly that newcomers to the field of regional anaesthesia familiarise themselves with the contents of Section 1 before attempting any practical technique. Section 1 PRINCIPLES AND PRACTICE contains an outline of the benefits of regional anaesthesia and our philosophy of its application. Most importantly for the novice, details on hazards, safety and precautions for safeguarding patient welfare are included. We make no apologies for stressing the need for resuscitation skills and equipment, constant intravenous access (even in minor procedures) and a knowledge of the pharmacology of the drugs to be employed.

Having assured themselves of the necessary skill and knowledge, less experienced readers will find in Section 2 OPERATIVE SITE a useful recap on the nerve supply to areas of the body, incorporating applied anatomy and guidance as to which peripheral nerve blocks are suitable for certain listed operations. Section 2 builds in a logical manner from the lower limb to the abdomen, through the thorax to the upper limb, and ends with the head and neck. Readers will thus be able in advance of a surgical list to revise the nerve supply to a particular operative site and select suitable peripheral nerve blocks. Once a technique has been decided upon, that particular nerve block will be found in Section 3 TECHNIQUES.

Section 3 carries descriptions in words and diagrams of each peripheral nerve block and can be directly accessed from the index of techniques in Section 4 if so desired. Note that for consistency, the right-sided approach has always been used. Each technique is accompanied by line and perspective diagrams to maximise the chance of success for the inexperienced. This volume is a distillation of our teaching and practice of regional anaesthesia but it should not be used as a substitute for direct supervision by an experienced mentor. Inexperienced practitioners should seek expert advice especially if attempting complex techniques. Suggested drugs and volumes of solution have been given after each technique but readers must be aware that these are only guidelines (based on a standard 70 kg patient). Although bupivacaine has been used most frequently in the drug boxes to illustrate the maximum duration of effect, shorter-acting agents may be clinically indicated in some situations. Onset times have been chosen to give an average time to onset of surgical anaesthesia and duration figures demonstrate the likely duration of an accurately placed block. Volume and dose must be modified in the light of actual patient size and morphology. Maximum dose guidelines must always be followed.

Section 4 REFERENCE has been incorporated for the benefit of those wishing to read more widely around the subject. The areas of the body are listed in a manner similar to Sections 2 and 3 and we have used popular regional anaesthesia sources (and some journal entries where necessary) to provide the reference material. An index of specific techniques is included for those experienced readers seeking direct access to an individual nerve block.

Principles and practice

Drug nomenclature

Throughout this volume the international non-proprietary name (INN) convention of the World Health Organisation has been applied. For the benefit of readers, alternative names of agents to which reference has been frequently made are listed in Table 1.1

Table 1.1 Drug nomenclature and alternative names

INN	Alternative name(s)
bupivacaine	marcaine, sensorcaine, carbostesin
chloroprocaine	2-chloroprocaine, nesacaine
lidocaine	xylocaine, lignocaine
prilocaine	citanest
procaine	novocaine
tetracaine	amethocaine
adrenaline	epinephrine
noradrenaline	norepinephrine
fentanyl	sublimaze
midazolam	hypnovel
thiopental	pentothal, thiopentone

Benefits of regional anaesthesia

Quality of analgesia

The mechanism of action of local anaesthetic agents is to reversibly inhibit sodium ion conductance across the nerve membrane. This has the effect of preventing depolarisation and onward neural transmission of noxious stimuli to the central neuraxis. This *prevention of nociception* distinguishes regional anaesthesia as a technique from globally acting analgesic drugs which affect the nociceptive pathway *after the stimulus has occurred*. As an example, opioids modulate the perception of pain at a central level whereas α_2-agonists alter the activity of nociceptive neurotransmitters in the spinal cord. Conversely, NSAIDs inhibit the sensitisation of peripheral pain receptors. The quality of analgesia which may be produced by regional anaesthesia is unsurpassed and particularly suited to the early post-operative period.

Duration of analgesia

The duration of analgesia can vary from a few hours to several days depending on the choice of agent, its concentration, the volume injected and the site of injection. Although major surgery may require post-operative analgesia for several days, many intermediate and minor surgical procedures have a relatively short duration of *severe* post-operative pain for which a few hours of intense analgesia are appropriate. Day case procedures fall into this category and respond well to peripheral nerve blocks of 3–6 hours duration enabling the patient to be discharged pain free without the risks associated with prolonged motor, sensory and proprioceptive dysfunction. For complex upper and lower limb surgery, bupivacaine 0.5% can be effective for up to 12 hours when used for major nerve and plexus blocks whilst bupivacaine 0.75% can produce in excess of 24 hours analgesia when used to block large peripheral nerves (for example, the sciatic or femoral nerves).

Insertion of catheters may enable a block to be extended for several days using either intermittent bolus injections or a continuous infusion. Continuous infusions provide a superior quality of analgesia with less haemodynamic disturbance. Additionally, there is less need for intervention by the nursing or medical staff, although occasional 'top up' boluses may be required to restore a regressing level of block. Until recently, the use of catheters has been restricted to the epidural route but the use of continuous catheter techniques for the perfusion of peripheral nerves is increasing.

Peri-operative use

Pain that occurs prior to surgery (for example, ischaemic rest pain, pain from gangrene or trauma) can be debilitating and complicates the management of the patient. The abolition of pain facilitates other aspects of care and optimises the patient's psychological state. Many patients with ischaemic leg changes suffer from diabetes mellitus and the presence of pain (often complicated by infection) destabilises both insulin requirement and metabolic balance. The use of large doses of opioids, to which the pain may be resistant, will often exacerbate the problems. In this situation, the pre-operative use of femoral and sciatic blockade (with catheters inserted into the nerve sheaths if possible) removes the need for opioid drugs and potentially improves diabetic management. The pre-operative use of either central neural blockade or peripheral nerve blocks to abolish pain in patients before undergoing limb amputation is of particular importance. Patients experiencing acute pain prior to undergoing amputation are likely to suffer from phantom limb pain post-operatively (up to 90% incidence in the first year) and the severity of the pain is generally a reflection of the pain experienced pre-operatively. If effective analgesia is established in the pre-operative period (using either epidural or peripheral nerve block) the incidence and severity of phantom limb pain can be markedly reduced.

Non-analgesic benefits

In addition to sensory and motor block, regional anaesthesia also produces autonomic block which can be of benefit. Blockade of the femoral and sciatic nerves produces a degree of unilateral vasodilatation which approximates to that produced by a lumbar epidural. This effect can be of value in the diagnosis and treatment of peripheral vascular disease. Post-operatively, the blood supply to the skin flaps and amputation stump is improved, resulting in optimum conditions for healing. Prolonged vasodilatation is desirable after vascular surgery when graft survival is improved. Brachial plexus anaesthesia will produce vasodilatation and improved perfusion and is thus indicated for trauma surgery (although the risk of obscuring compartment syndrome must be borne in mind) and the fashioning of arterio-venous fistulae.

Systemic benefits

The benefits of successful regional anaesthesia are not totally due to the relief of pain at the site of injury. The systemic effects of pain are widespread (Table 1.2). The consequences of ineffective treatment of pain are manifested in an increased risk of post-operative complications, slower recovery and delayed discharge. The systemic stress response, accompanied by a rise in circulating catecholamines and ACTH, may be triggered by severe pain resulting from any cause. Over the last decade, emphasis has been placed on the investigation of the ways in which different anaesthetic techniques can modify or abolish the stress response which has led to the concept of 'stress-free anaesthesia and surgery'. Despite initial uncertainty as to the importance of the stress response, it is now widely accepted that the complex neuro-endocrine, metabolic and immunological changes that occur after surgery have a detrimental effect on the myocardium, the respiratory system and the gastrointestinal tract.

Many studies have shown that neural blockade with local anaesthetic agents can be effective in abolishing the stress response. The relationship between good analgesia, the abolition of the stress response and a measurable improvement in outcome is complex and confusing. There is a lack of hard data from well conducted, randomised trials due largely to the difficulty of defining the goals to be achieved. The consensus is that properly managed regional anaesthetic techniques are the most effective way of providing post-operative analgesia for major surgery and offer the best available means of modifying the stress response to surgery and improving outcome.

Table 1.2 Major systemic effects of pain

System	Effects
cardiovascular	increased plasma catecholamines increased myocardial contractility tachycardia decreased organ perfusion
respiratory	reduced FRC reduced PEFR impaired cough basal airway collapse
gastrointestinal	reduced splanchnic perfusion increased secretions increased sphincter tone decreased motility gastric dilatation
renal	increased renin/aldosterone/ cortisol/vasopressin potassium loss water and sodium retention
metabolic	increased catabolism and nitrogen loss insulin resistance

Rational use of peripheral nerve blockade

Introduction

The successful use of regional anaesthesia requires sufficient initial enthusiasm to learn a wide variety of techniques. In the early stages of this phase, the accent is justifiably on acquiring the necessary skill to perform the blocks safely and successfully. At a later stage, it becomes important to consider how these newly acquired skills can be incorporated into clinical practice to the benefit of the patient throughout the entire peri-operative period. Experience is required both to select the correct technique (or combination of techniques) and to learn how to care for the patient who is undergoing surgery 'under local'. If the potential benefits of regional anaesthesia are to be made available to the patient, the clinician responsible for initiating the technique must realise that injecting the local anaesthetic drug and confirming that the block is working marks only the beginning of the patient's care. Managing the conscious patient while surgery is being carried out requires organisation and attention to detail if the patient is not to regret the decision to stay awake during their operation.

Anatomical considerations

The main prerequisite for successful regional anaesthesia is a full understanding of the relevant topographical landmarks, the intervening structures between the skin and the target nerve(s) and the course and immediate relations of the target nerve(s). Each peripheral nerve usually has a cutaneous sensory component and a somatic component supplying motor fibres to muscles and sensory and proprioceptive fibres to joints and other deep structures.

GENERAL PRINCIPLES OF PERIPHERAL NERVE ANATOMY

- Cutaneous sensory distribution can be mapped either as an individual dermatome which represents single nerve root derivation or as a peripheral nerve territory which represents derivation from multiple nerve roots.
- If a local anaesthetic block is performed at the level of the nerve roots (such as an

interscalene brachial plexus block) the onset of anaesthesia is best monitored by checking the dermatomal pattern of anaesthesia. Any failure or inadequacy will usually manifest itself in a dermatomal pattern but if the technique is performed at the level of a peripheral nerve, then failure will occur in the distribution of the nerve territory. A knowledge of the limits of territory is therefore necessary.

- The deep structures supplied by the nerve do not necessarily underlie the cutaneous distribution. The musculocutaneous nerve (C5, 6, 7), for example, supplies the flexor muscles in the upper arm but its cutaneous distribution is in the forearm (the lateral cutaneous nerve of forearm). This difference between the motor and sensory components of a nerve block can be utilised to allow the patient to make voluntary muscle movement during surgery. Thus, surgery for Dupuytren's contracture can be undertaken after blocking the ulnar and median nerves at the wrist to produce sensory block in the surgical field but still allow the patient to flex the forearm muscles which remain unaffected.

- Hilton's law states that the motor nerve to a muscle tends to give a branch of supply to the joint which the muscle moves and another branch to the skin over the joint. Generally, this means that the nerve supply to a joint is derived from all the nerves which traverse that joint. This principle is important in planning procedures for joint surgery. In the knee, for example, the obturator, femoral, sciatic and lateral cutaneous nerve of thigh all contribute fibres to the internal structures and need to be blocked in varying combinations, depending on the type of surgery planned.

Surgical considerations

Successful regional anaesthesia requires careful choice of which nerves to anaesthetise and this depends on an understanding of the surgeon's intentions. In turn, the surgeon must understand the different operating conditions that regional anaesthesia provides and be prepared to modify the surgical technique if necessary.

SURGICAL CONSIDERATIONS

- The site of the surgical incision should be carefully considered because it may cross the territory of several adjacent nerves. Even if the incision is entirely within the normal territory of a single nerve, it is prudent to block adjacent nerve territories as they are very variable and may have considerable overlap. Surgically, the operation may also turn out to be more extensive than first planned.

- The site of limb surgery affects pre-operative planning. Proximal surgery above the knee or elbow usually requires plexus anaesthesia which is of shorter duration than discrete nerve blocks (more appropriate for distal surgery). However, even when the surgery is distal, surgical needs may dictate that a tourniquet is necessary and this may demand a plexus block in order to enable the patient to tolerate the tourniquet.

- Surgical stimulation may cause the patient distress despite a fully functioning block. This commonly occurs during hernia or scrotal surgery when traction on the spermatic cord causes deep visceral pain in the abdomen despite a satisfactory somatic block. It is vital that the surgeon is fully aware of the limitations of regional anaesthesia in this situation and modifies the surgical technique accordingly.

Patient selection

Indications

Regional anaesthesia in the conscious patient requires active cooperation. In patients where this is not forthcoming, as may occur with intoxication, head injuries or severe anxiety, general anaesthesia (or cautious intravenous sedation) supplemented by a regional technique is the most sensible course. For most patients a brief outline of the benefits of regional anaesthesia (pain relief of several hours duration, less nausea, less drowsiness and an earlier promise of a cup of tea) usually results in a willing patient and overcomes reluctance of 'needling'. No patient should be coerced into a regional technique against their will. Children present specific problems. The older child will usually cooperate, especially if EMLA cream is used to make skin penetration painless. Reluctant children and those too young to understand the procedure will require general anaesthesia, although the opportunity should be taken to provide post-operative analgesia by the use of an appropriate regional anaesthetic technique.

Contraindications

The preparation of a patient for major surgery under regional anaesthesia is similar to that for general anaesthesia. If the patient is not appropriately fit for general anaesthesia, then a regional technique is not necessarily a suitable alternative. Correctable pathophysiological disturbance should be investigated and treated before instituting regional anaesthesia which must not be regarded as a 'short cut' or less demanding alternative.

There are relatively few specific contraindications to regional anaesthesia and most are only relative in that whilst, for instance, infection or trauma over the site of the proposed block may prevent one technique, a more proximal or distal combination of blocks is often possible.

CONTRAINDICATIONS TO REGIONAL ANAESTHESIA

- patient refusal despite full discussions
- psychiatric or psychological disturbance
- full anticoagulation or coagulopathy
- infection overlying the site of injection
- trauma/burns over site of injection
- pre-existing neurological deficit
- uncorrected metabolic derangement

Management

Pre-operative management

Having decided to use regional anaesthesia, it is essential that the implications and effects are discussed fully with the patient. Whilst complications are rare and largely avoidable, side effects such as motor, autonomic and proprioceptive dysfunction may worry the patient unless they are prepared in advance. Minor side effects such as stinging from the initial injection of the local anaesthetic solution or the paraesthesiae that accompany the onset

and offset of the block need to be discussed with the patient. The possibility of motor weakness that outlasts the return of sensation should also be emphasised.

The variety of sensations that the patient might experience during surgery despite a fully functioning block should be fully explained to prevent them from being interpreted as a sign of failed anaesthesia. Feelings of pressure and tension are common but should not cause distress. Disordered temperature sensation may alarm the patient if cold fluids are applied to the wound site. A variety of non-specific sensations which are painless but nonetheless disconcerting may be felt. Reassurance that this is normal and not a sign of a failed technique is necessary to maintain patient confidence. The analogy of local anaesthesia in the dentist's chair usually helps to explain the perception of extraneous sensations.

The decision about whether to use regional anaesthesia alone or to combine it with general anaesthesia must be made at the pre-operative visit and fully explored. It is important to explain to the patient the likely effects of the motor and sensory loss that will last into the post-operative period. This avoids the patient misinterpreting the apparent loss of part of their anatomy during their early post-operative recovery. Light general anaesthesia is easier and safer to manage offering quicker recovery than several boluses of intravenous sedation which may become necessary during surgery if the patient becomes uncooperative. Post-operative sedation may be marked, especially if a benzodiazepine has been administered peri-operatively. Indications for combining general and regional anaesthesia are listed in the chart.

INDICATIONS FOR COMBINING GENERAL AND REGIONAL ANAESTHESIA

- patient preference
- surgical technique – if surgery causes reflex stimuli outside area of anaesthesia e.g. traction on spermatic cord during herniorrhaphy under field block
- prolonged operation – beyond 1 hour; many patients find it very uncomfortable to lie still for over an hour
- tourniquet pain
- amputations
- cancer surgery

Premedication

The use of premedication for patients undergoing regional anaesthesia is subject to the same guidelines that apply to general anaesthesia. Many patients are happy to avoid any sedation and clouding of consciousness following an adequate explanation of what to expect, whilst others prefer to know little of the actual surgery. Much will depend on the skills and confidence of the person performing the technique. Where premedication is prescribed, the patient must remain able to cooperate during the regional technique; therefore, heavy sedation should be avoided.

Pre-operative starvation

A patient who is to receive regional anaesthesia should undergo the same protocol of pre-operative restriction of fluids and food as patients undergoing the same procedure under general anaesthesia. Sudden loss of consciousness can occur for a number of reasons during the conduct of regional anaesthesia. The patient is, therefore, exposed to the same risks of regurgitation or vomiting as during general anaesthesia. Starvation is essential in the event that inadequate anaesthesia requires supplementation with general anaesthesia.

Performing the technique

All regional techniques are capable of causing complications. Local anaesthetic drugs have potentially serious toxic properties. No patient should undergo regional anaesthesia unless the operator is fully trained in the recognition of complications and is competent to treat them. Full resuscitation facilities must be immediately available together with suitable patient monitoring equipment.

Safe conduct of regional anaesthesia requires suitable surroundings of cleanliness and space with a good source of ambient light and warmth with adequate privacy for the patient. An assistant trained in anaesthesia and recovery procedures and familiar with regional anaesthesia is an invaluable help to both doctor and patient.

If the patient is comfortable and correctly positioned and the operator is comfortable and well prepared, then the chances of the technique being performed quickly and successfully are increased. The equipment, sterile towels and drugs required for the procedure should be available and checked before the patient is positioned. The bed or trolley should be adjusted to the correct height for the operator and the patient positioned comfortably and accurately, using pillows and other supports as indicated. The assistant can help the patient to maintain the correct position and will often provide psychological support and reassurance, allowing the clinician to concentrate on the procedure. Once the technique is started, conversation should be restricted to informing the patient what to expect next, with reassurance as necessary. If an explanation of the technique is being given to observers, then the patient must be informed so that they do not misinterpret remarks. Explanations given in the presence of a conscious patient must take into account the patient's situation and understanding.

Where local anaesthesia is to be combined with general anaesthesia, some authorities advocate performing the blocks with the patient awake on the grounds of avoiding inadvertent intraneural injection. However, the majority of children receive their local anaesthetic block after induction of general anaesthesia without evidence of an increased risk of neural damage. In adults, many techniques such as intercostal, interpleural, caudal and femoral and sciatic nerve blocks are traditionally performed after induction of anaesthesia without demonstrable extra risk. Provided that appropriate care is taken to avoid intraneural and intravascular injection, most regional techniques can be performed under general anaesthesia if necessary. Epidural injections above the cauda equina and the interscalene approach to the brachial plexus are safer when performed on conscious patients.

Testing the block

After allowing a suitable period for the onset of analgesia, the success of a block can be tested with pinprick (using a 21 G needle) and loss of muscle power. Although formal dermatomal loss of sensation can be tested, the prime requirement is loss of sensation of superficial and deep structures in the region of the operative site. The ultimate test is successful completion of the operation without patient discomfort. Testing should be noted on the anaesthetic record.

Peri-operative management

To the conscious patient, the operating theatre can be a hostile and intimidating environment and all staff should be aware of the noise and other disturbances they make. Every step of the preparation and positioning of the patient should be explained and directed towards making the patient comfortable and confident. On no account should any preparations for surgery begin until the patient is confident in the quality of the anaesthesia. Resist the temptation to repeatedly question the patient as to what they can feel – instead tell them what to expect as the block develops, ask them to say when the different stages happen and use objective tests of motor and sensory loss in the area of the block to decide on the adequacy of the analgesia.

Dissuade the surgeon from saying 'Can you feel this?' or 'Does this hurt?' as they make the incision. Remind the patient of the sensations that were discussed during the pre-operative visit.

If significant motor weakness occurs, the affected part must be properly protected from hyperextension injury due to unrestrained movement. The lack of sensory perception requires that the relevant pressure points are well protected during surgery. Once the operation is underway and much of the noise of preparation subsides, many patients will drift off to sleep if they are comfortable and have been premedicated. Others prefer to have a gentle conversation or even watch their procedure on screen which the increasing use of video technology makes possible.

Recording the block (documentation)

There is no substitute for accurate record keeping. Regional anaesthesia is no exception to this rule. The authors recommend the recording of the following: technique, approach, type of needle, use of nerve stimulator (or not), the agent, its concentration and volume (including vasoconstrictor). The occurrence of any paraesthesiae, bleeding or other sequelae of the injection should also be noted.

Post-operative care

The degree of supervision required post-operatively depends on the anticipated duration and the extent of the block. For day case,

outpatient and emergency department surgery, the prime requirement is early discharge of the patient suitably able to care for themself. To achieve this aim, nerve blockade should be as peripheral as possible and of short duration rather than proximal plexus blocks of long duration. There are inherent risks associated with flail limbs – the arm is an important part of balance and self-protection and the leg is clearly fundamental to weight bearing. The patient should not be discharged without evidence that motor block has fully regressed and that the patient can self-care. If for any reason the limb is still affected by a block at the time of discharge, it should either be immobilised in a sling for protection or the patient must remain non-weight bearing during the journey home and instructed to rest until full function returns.

For inpatients undergoing major surgery, long duration of analgesia is a benefit, provided that due regard is paid to the specific care of the anaesthetised area. Patients who have undergone lower limb blocks or lumbar plexus blockade must only be mobilised under direct supervision until they can demonstrate full motor and sensory recovery by the ability to fully flex and extend the hip and knee against resistance (motor) and have normal proprioception and sensation in the great toe (sensory). Some authorities recommend testing perianal skin sensation to ensure complete sacral nerve root recovery but in practice this is not always necessary. The upper limb must be properly immobilised with a sling or other support until full function returns. Any patient who has long-lasting cutaneous analgesia should be encouraged to move the affected limb in order to prevent pressure sores developing on the dependent areas. Use of lower limb blocks may require antithrombotic precautions until mobilisation.

Ischaemic pain

Plaster casts, compression dressings or limb splints can cause vascular inadequacy and ischaemia if incorrectly applied. The early swelling and discolouration that ensues should alert attending staff to remove the dressing and examine the limb even though the patient may not complain of pain. Similarly, compartment syndrome following closed trauma to a limb can cause major ischaemic damage if unrecognised in the early stages. In patients who have functioning nerve blockade, pain may be absent until the late stages of ischaemia, although it may break through a block in the same way as pathological pain breaks through functioning epidural blockade. Nursing and medical staff involved in the care of patients with peripheral nerve blockade must understand the implications of prolonged analgesia and modify their care accordingly.

Further analgesic requirements

For many minor and intermediate surgical procedures, a long-acting discrete nerve block may provide all the analgesia that the patient needs. For more painful procedures, a course of compound oral analgesics or non-steroidal anti-inflammatory agents may be required when normal sensation returns. Patients should be instructed to start oral analgesia before the effects of the nerve block wear off completely in order to ensure that the analgesia remains continuous. Pain outside the anaesthetised area or breakthrough pain in the immediate post-operative period may need parenteral opioids which can also provide a general sedative effect in patients who have good analgesia but are restless due to other stimuli. It is most important to achieve and maintain good quality analgesia from the outset and to supplement the regional technique as necessary until the patient is comfortable.

Equipment

General anaesthesia and resuscitation

Local anaesthetic drugs are hazardous due to their cardiovascular and neurological toxicity if administered intravascularly or in excess. The practice of regional anaesthesia demands proficiency at airway management and cardio-respiratory resuscitation. Local anaesthetic agents should not be administered to a patient without the immediate availability of intravenous therapy, suction, cardiorespiratory resuscitation equipment and monitoring facilities, and preferably full general anaesthesia back up.

Supplementary requirements

With the exception of a peripheral nerve stimulator (PNS), peripheral nerve blocks require few specialised items. All techniques should be performed with sterile (preferably disposable) items and the preparation of drugs and equipment should be undertaken in conditions of good light on a surface of adequate size so that sterility can be maintained and equipment suitably arranged. The choice of commercially available packs suitable for regional anaesthesia or packs produced within the hospital is a matter of local requirements and financial comparisons. Solutions used to sterilise skin should not be replaced on the sterile surface but should be disposed of before the local anaesthetic solution is drawn up to avoid any potential confusion. Sterile surgical gloves should be worn and a rigid no touch technique applied. For complex techniques (such as the placement of catheters) use full sterile precautions.

The 'immobile needle', described by Winnie (1969), uses a short (10–20 cm) extension tube to isolate the needle from movements of the syringe during aspiration, injection and syringe exchange, thus minimising the risks of nerve trauma and needle misplacement. It also allows the operator to use both hands to perform the technique and an assistant to make the injections.

Needles
Infiltration

Preliminary skin weals and infiltration techniques are performed with fine gauge (23 G or 25 G) hypodermic needles. For infiltration over a wider area, use spinal needles of similar gauge.

Choice of tip

The nomenclature and bevel angle of standard hypodermic needles are determined by British Standard (BS) 5081 Pt 2 (1987). So-called 'long' bevelled needles have a bevel cut at 12°(±2°). Short bevelled needles have no equivalent BS and the bevel may be cut between 18° and 45°, the facets being ground so that the needle parts tissue rather than cutting it. Short bevel needles offer more resistance during insertion and thus more feedback to the operator. Figure 1.1 shows the overall dimensions and bevel angles of the tip of a typical short bevelled needle. The 'security' bead near the junction of the shaft and the hub was originally necessary to prevent migration and loss of the shaft if the hub broke off due to fatigue of the solder used to join both parts. Modern needles are made from surgical stainless steel with very secure hubs, thus the bead is now redundant although it may be used as an attachment for the alligator clip of a PNS.

There continues to be disagreement and uncertainty about the design of the needle tip and its effect on the incidence of nerve trauma following regional anaesthesia. Work by Selander et al (1977) showed that both in vivo and in vitro, short bevel needles cause less damage to nerves and are associated with a lower incidence of neuritis although this view has been challenged by Rice & McMahon (1992) who showed that the reverse was true (albeit in a rat sciatic nerve model). Nevertheless, it is clear that there are no clinical data to support the suggestions that needle tip design and the elicitation of paraesthesiae have a direct link with the incidence of neuropathy (Moore et al 1994). Other research has suggested that needles without any bevel at all would be logical and pencil point needles have been designed to prevent neural damage. Pencil point needles are designed with a side port to prevent intraneural injection, although in a number of studies it has been shown that intraneural, as opposed to epineural, injection is most unlikely and difficult to reproduce in vitro.

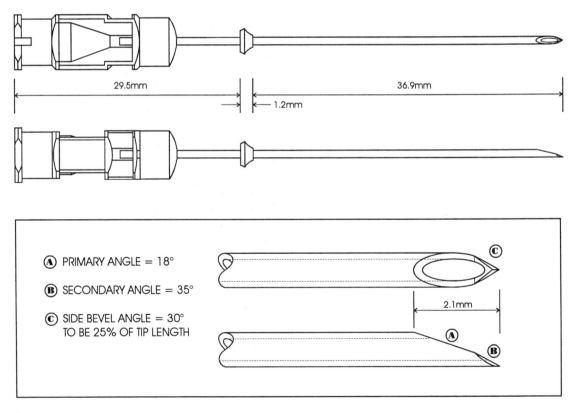

Fig 1.1
Regional block needle (reproduced with permission from Becton Dickinson UK Ltd)

Despite the controversy surrounding the choice of needle tip, short bevel or pencil point needles are strongly recommended for major nerve blockade because the amount of feedback from them is so superior to long bevelled needles that the likelihood of success is enhanced.

Peripheral nerve stimulator (PNS)

Low power electrical stimuli have been used to locate peripheral nerves since 1912 although it is only in recent years that modern electronics have made it possible to design safe, practical and portable PNSs for routine clinical use. There is debate about the ideal characteristics for a PNS and there are very few commercially available units that satisfy all theoretical requirements. Figure 1.2 shows the most recent version of a popular model. The ideal characteristics of a PNS are listed in the chart.

For a full explanation of the electrical theory of nerve stimulation, readers are directed to the review of Pither et al (1985). The PNS can be used to electrolocate any peripheral nerve of mixed motor and sensory function. Whilst a purely sensory nerve can be stimulated at high power to produce paraesthesiae, this is an unreliable method that may be painful for the patient and is not recommended.

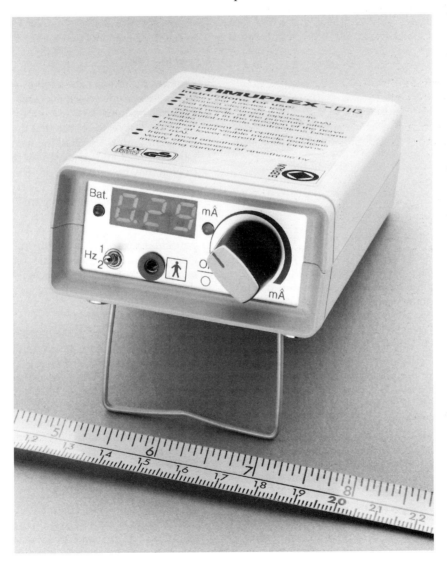

Fig 1.2
A peripheral nerve stimulator (reproduced with permission from Braun UK)

IDEAL CHARACTERISTICS OF A PNS

- Portable, battery operated, with detachable and sterilisable leads
- Clearly marked electrodes indicating that the cathode (–ve) is attached to the needle
- Universal alligator-type terminals for use with a wide variety of needles
- Digital display of delivered current (and/or voltage) with linear output; below 1 mA, sensitivity increased to allow precise current readings
- Voltage (9 V) and current (5 mA) limited to cope with variable resistance of body tissues
- Short duration impulse (less than 100 μsec) at frequency of 1–2 Hz so that motor nerves are stimulated preferentially to sensory nerves

Note. The product of mA and μsec is nanocoulombs (nC) and the digital readout of a PNS can be calibrated in nC. For example, 1 mA × 100 μsec = 100 nC which is sufficient charge to stimulate a nerve if the needle is within 2–3 mm.

Indications

The PNS is not a substitute for inadequate anatomical knowledge and should not be employed to hunt blindly for nerves; it is used to best advantage when confirming accurate placement of a needle tip close to, but not touching the required nerve. The PNS is most useful in the location of deeply placed nerves and plexuses which have a characteristic distribution of muscle movement when stimulated and which are traditionally associated with a low incidence of success when the technique is attempted 'blind'. The PNS may also be appropriate for accurately locating a particular part of a large nerve or plexus when the anaesthetic requirements demand that a specific branch of the nerve be blocked, e.g. the deep division of the femoral nerve which supplies the sensory fibres of the knee joint and the motor supply to the quadriceps femoris and the patellar mechanism. The distinct end point of pulse synchronous muscle movement that accompanies nerve location makes the PNS a valuable aid to learning peripheral nerve blocks

and similarly allows nerve location in patients who are sedated or anaesthetised. Approaches that benefit from the use of a PNS are shown in the chart.

APPROACHES THAT BENEFIT FROM USE OF A PNS

- All approaches to brachial plexus
- Suprascapular nerve
- Radial nerve at the elbow
- Median nerve at the elbow
- All approaches to sciatic nerve
- Femoral nerve (including '3 in 1')
- Obturator nerve
- Popliteal fossa block

Using the PNS

1. Connect the anode (+ve lead) to a large ground electrode which is placed under the patient's body well away from the site of needle insertion to ensure that the current flows through the path of the nerve. Test the battery power and check circuit integrity (which may be an audible or visual signal depending on the model of PNS) and set delivered current at a moderate level, 3 mA for example.
2. Use a standard approach to the nerve, paying particular regard to the tactile information being generated by the needle. Advance the needle until within the expected vicinity of the nerve. Attach the cathode (–ve lead) to the needle hub.
3. *Turn on the stimulator.*
4. When using current of the order of 3 mA or less, the nerve will not be stimulated if the needle tip is more than 1 cm distant. Coulomb's law (inverse square law) implies that the power needed to stimulate a nerve increases very quickly as the distance from the needle tip to the nerve increases. Painful levels of stimulation may be needed if the nerve is more than 2 cm distant. Thus, pulse synchronous movement with low power levels indicate that the needle is close to the nerve. In order to place the needle tip adjacent to the nerve, carefully adjust the needle tip position whilst reducing the stimulus strength until the muscle movement is just discernible with the minimum stimulus possible (usually 0.1–0.5 mA delivered current). A sudden increase in

muscle movement or the onset of pain indicates that the needle is in direct contact with the nerve and it should be withdrawn slightly before the injection. The minimum stimulating current and voltage will vary according to which nerve is being blocked, the age of the patient and the presence of neuropathy. Small, superficial nerves such as the median or radial require 0.1–0.3 mA and less than 1 V while large, deep nerves such as the sciatic or obturator require up to 2 mA and up to 3 V. In the elderly or in the presence of neuropathy greater stimulus strength will be necessary.

5 Having located the nerve, immobilise the needle and aspirate gently. An initial injection of 1–2 ml may produce an *increased muscle movement* as the local anaesthetic improves the electrical conductivity, usually followed quickly by a *fade in the movements* which can be attributed to the nerve being displaced by the injection and thus increasing the needle–nerve distance. There should be neither resistance to flow nor pain on injection, either of which can indicate subperineural or intraneural needle placement. If the patient is sedated or anaesthetised, pain or paraesthesiae on injection will not be apparent, so extreme care must be taken to avoid neural damage. Any resistance to injection must be assumed to indicate incorrect needle position which requires adjustment aided by the PNS so that the needle is still in close proximity to the nerve but the injection of local anaesthetic solution is of low resistance.

Insulated versus uninsulated needles

There is no consensus amongst PNS users as to whether the type of needle used is important in the success of the block or the risk of neural damage. A number of theories have been advanced to support both types of needle but without firm evidence to confirm any clinical benefit. From a practical perspective, uninsulated needles are widely available in a greater variety of length and diameter and are cheaper than insulated needles. For many peripheral nerve blocks uninsulated needles are entirely satisfactory with little loss of current along the length of the shaft. However, for deep nerves where the needle has to traverse a large muscle mass, e.g. the anterior approach to the sciatic nerve, the radial nerve (at the elbow) and the suprascapular nerve, insulated needles are recommended because they avoid localised direct stimulation of the muscles through which the needle passes. This direct stimulation can cause confusion about nerve location and requires up to twice the stimulus strength that insulated needles require.

Local anaesthetic drugs

Introduction

Any drug which possesses membrane stabilising properties has the potential for use as a local anaesthetic agent. This fact explains the local anaesthetic effects of drugs such as disopyramide and practolol under experimental conditions. Clinically useful local anaesthetic agents fall into two groups, esters and amides, based on their chemical structure. The structure of local anaesthetic agents is three part and consists of an aromatic ring linked by an intermediate chain to an amino group. The intermediate chain may contain an ester or amide linkage, hence their classification as esters or amides. The two groups show differences in their physicochemical properties.

Esters

Ester local anaesthetic agents have an esteric bond (–COO–) between aromatic and amino components. As the esteric bond is relatively unstable these solutions are liable to degradation and thus are disadvantaged by a relatively short shelf life. Esters are hydrolysed in the plasma by pseudocholinesterase which renders them comparatively non toxic but also of short duration. Ester local anaesthetic agents in clinical use include procaine, amethocaine and chloroprocaine.

Amides

Amides have a much stronger intermediate bond (–NHCO–) than the esters. They are, therefore, stable in solution and little affected by changes in pH (as may occur in adrenaline-containing mixtures) and are suitable for heat sterilisation, in contrast to esters. Amide local anaesthetic agents (for example, lidocaine) do not undergo plasma hydrolysis but are liver metabolised usually by a combination of oxidative dealkylation and hydroxylation.

Mechanism of action

Both esters and amides act in a similar manner to cause a reversible interruption to the conduction of impulses along nerve fibres. Propagation of an impulse along a nerve is caused by a sequence of depolarisation and repolarisation passing along the nerve fibre. In the resting state nerve fibres display polarisation, that is to say sodium is present in greater concentration outside the cell than in, and potassium in greater concentration inside the cell than out. The mechanism of action causing depolarisation is a flow of sodium ions through specific sodium channels (which exist like pores in the phospholipid membrane) from the outside to the inside of the nerve fibre. A flow of potassium ions in the reverse direction results in repolarisation. Ionic pumps restore the balance of ionic composition after repolarisation.

The precise mode of action of local anaesthetic drugs is not completely understood but the cardinal feature appears to be an inhibition of the increase in membrane permeability to sodium ions thus preventing depolarisation. This effect is mediated by preventing the sodium channels from opening and hence the membrane is stabilised and the resting polarised state is maintained.

Physicochemical factors

Local anaesthetic agents generally possess poor solubility in water. Most commercial preparations consist of a salt (usually the hydrochloride which is water soluble) and after injection this is subject to ionisation of a variable degree, depending on pK_a, to produce a local anaesthetic anion and a chloride cation. The anion further dissociates at body pH to a hydrogen ion and free local anaesthetic base. The free base is lipid soluble and penetrates the epineurium, which is a lipid bilayer, after which ionisation occurs in the water-based axoplasm and the ionic form is then able to reach and affect the sodium channels within the nerve fibre itself. As the effect grows in magnitude, conduction is first slowed and then later prevented entirely.

The pK_a of a drug is the pH at which it is 50% ionised and 50% un-ionised. Most local anaesthetic agents have pK_a values greater than 7.4 and the greater the pK_a, the less the amount of free base at body pH.

As it is only the un-ionised form that can penetrate the nerve membrane, pK_a has a profound effect on speed of onset. The lower the pK_a, the faster the onset of effect will be.

Potency of local anaesthetic drugs is largely determined by lipid solubility. The higher the lipid/water partition coefficient, the greater the potency of the agent. The degree of protein binding affects duration of action of local anaesthetic drugs. Agents which posses a high degree of protein binding attach more strongly to their active sites in the nerve membrane and thus have a prolonged duration of action. A comparison of physicochemical properties for the more common local anaesthetic drugs is shown in Table 1.3.

Individual agents

Lidocaine HCl

Rapid onset and medium duration. Available as the following solutions for injection (anhydrous):

0.5% containing lidocaine hydrochloride
  5 mg/ml
1% containing lidocaine hydrochloride
  10 mg/ml
2% containing lidocaine hydrochloride
  20 mg/ml
0.5% containing lidocaine hydrochloride
  5 mg/ml plus adrenaline 5 µg/ml
1% containing lidocaine hydrochloride
  10 mg/ml plus adrenaline 5 µg/ml
2% containing lidocaine hydrochloride
  20 mg/ml plus adrenaline 5 µg/ml

    The concentrations of adrenaline in the above solutions represent 1 in 200 000 dilution.
    Sodium chloride is added to these solutions to achieve isotonicity. Inactive ingredients are the preservatives sodium metabisulphite and methylparahydroxybenzoate.
    Lidocaine is also available for dental use plain or mixed with adrenaline or noradrenaline and in various preparations for topical use. Lidocaine is one of the constituents of EMLA cream.
    Maximum recommended dose in adults (data sheet) 200 mg.

> Note. Due to enzyme inhibition, cimetidine may impair the metabolism of lidocaine.

Bupivacaine HCl

Slow onset and long duration. Available as the following solutions for injection (anhydrous):

0.25% containing bupivacaine hydrochloride
  2.5 mg/ml
0.5% containing bupivacaine hydrochloride
  5 mg/ml
0.75% containing bupivacaine hydrochloride
  7.5 mg/ml (contraindicated in obstetric use).
0.25% containing bupivacaine hydrochloride
  2.5 mg/ml plus adrenaline 5.5 µg/ml
0.5% containing bupivacaine hydrochloride
  5 mg/ml plus adrenaline 5.5 µg/ml

    The concentrations of adrenaline in the above solutions represent 1 in 200 000 dilution.
    Sodium chloride is added to these solutions to achieve isotonicity. Adrenaline containing solutions also contain sodium metabisulphite.

Table 1.3 Physicochemical properties of local anaesthetic agents

Agent	Molecular weight	pK_a (25 °C)	Partition coefficient	Protein binding %
Esters				
procaine	236	8.9	0.02	5.8
amethocaine	264	8.5	4.1	76
chloroprocaine	271	8.7	0.14	–
Amides				
prilocaine	220	7.9	0.9	55
lidocaine	234	7.9	2.9	64
mepivacaine	246	7.6	0.8	78
bupivacaine	288	8.1	27.5	96
ropivacaine	274	8.0	27.5	95

Maximum recommended single dose for adult 150 mg. Dosage should not exceed 2 mg/kg.

Available as a solution for spinal anaesthesia containing: Bupivacaine hydrochloride anhydrous 5 mg/ml plus dextrose anhydrous 72.2 mg/ml. Specific gravity 1.026 at 20 °C.

Ropivacaine

Ropivacaine is a new amide due to be released in the near future. Ropivacaine is structurally similar to both bupivacaine and mepivacaine. Early work suggests that ropivacaine may have a similar profile to bupivacaine with less risk of cardiotoxicity.

Prilocaine HCl

Medium onset and medium duration. Low toxicity compared with other agents. May cause methaemoglobinaemia if dosage exceeds 600 mg. Available as the following solutions for injection (anhydrous):

0.5% containing prilocaine hydrochloride
    5 mg/ml
1% containing prilocaine hydrochloride
    10 mg/ml
2% containing prilocaine hydrochloride
    20 mg/ml

    Also available for dental use as:

4% containing prilocaine hydrochloride
    40 mg/ml
3% containing prilocaine hydrochloride
    30 mg/ml plus felypressin 0.03 unit/ml

The above solutions contain sodium chloride to achieve isotonicity. The 4% solution contains sodium hydroxide and multidose vials contain methylparahydroxybenzoate as preservative.

Maximum dose in healthy adults 400 mg.

Other agents

Amethocaine is a useful agent for topical application. It is rapidly absorbed from mucous membranes and should be used with care due to its relatively toxic nature. **Benzocaine** is an agent of low potency and toxicity used in throat lozenges. **Cocaine** is an ester which readily penetrates mucous membranes and is used in ENT procedures because of its intense vasoconstrictor effect. It is highly toxic and should not be given parenterally. **Procaine** is an ester of slow onset and short duration seldom used today but previously employed for spinal anaesthesia. **Mepivacaine** is an amide of rapid onset and medium duration somewhat less toxic than lidocaine. It is not available in the UK. **Chloroprocaine** is an ester of rapid onset and short duration. It is relatively non-toxic due to plasma hydrolysis. Pharmacological comparison between agents is given in Table 1.4.

Table 1.4 Pharmacological properties of local anaesthetic drugs

Agent	Onset	Relative potency	Duration
procaine	slow	1	short
chloroprocaine	rapid	1	short
amethocaine	slow	8	long
prilocaine	rapid	2	medium
lidocaine	rapid	2	medium
bupivacaine	medium	8	long
ropivacaine	medium	8	long

Complications of regional anaesthesia

Introduction

Complications of peripheral neural blockade are uncommon provided that reasonable care is exercised in assessing the patient so that unsuitable patients are excluded and patient management is appropriate both during and after surgery. Complications range from the trivial to the life threatening and may be related to the block technique, the local anaesthetic used or the selection and management of the patient (Table 1.5). Some complications are common to all blocks whilst others are specific to a particular technique.

Table 1.5 Complications of regional anaesthesia

Technique	Patient	Drug
neural damage	pre-existing neural pathology	intravascular injection
haematoma	inappropriate sedation	drug overdose
pneumothorax	vasovagal faint	anaphylactoid reaction
widespread block	faulty positioning tourniquet pressure compartment syndrome	excess vasoconstriction 'wrong' solution methaemo-globinaemia

Complications of the technique
Neurological damage

Nerve damage is often cited by clinicians to explain their reluctance to perform peripheral regional anaesthesia. This belies the very low incidence of neurological damage directly attributable to needle damage (0.36–1.9% incidence most studies). The great majority of post-operative neurological sequelae are temporary and are typically sensory dysaesthesiae within the distribution of the blocked nerve or one of its branches; recovery is within days to a few weeks. Neurological damage in patients undergoing general anaesthesia alone has been reported due to faulty positioning of the patient, surgical retraction and other unrelated causes. The femoral, ulnar, peroneal, lateral cutaneous nerve of thigh and the brachial plexus are at risk of compression due to over extension or flexion, and inadequate padding during prolonged surgery.

The most common injury is neuropraxia, where the nerve remains anatomically intact but individual nerve axons or bundles are functionally disrupted. Direct laceration by the needle tip is probably the most frequent cause of nerve damage. Other important and avoidable causes are: firstly, compression by hydraulic pressure within a rigid compartment, e.g. the ulnar nerve in the sulcus of the medial epicondyle of the humerus, and secondly, over extension or flexion of limbs for prolonged periods.

The ideal needle is the subject of debate (p. 10). Current opinion still supports the use of short bevelled needles for all discrete nerve blocks to increase the feedback during nerve location and reduce the likelihood of intraneural needle placement. It is important to minimise the use of paraesthesiae as an aid to locating a nerve (using a PNS obviates the need to seek paraesthesiae).

Haematoma formation

Many peripheral nerves run in close proximity to major vessels and inadvertent vascular puncture is a constant risk. In addition to the toxic effects of intravascular injection, extravasation and haematoma formation may distort local anatomical landmarks thus adding to the difficulty of nerve location and complicating the surgical approach. Other factors include increased patient discomfort, neural compression and subsequent neurological sequelae. If the patient has disordered clotting, the risks of such a complication must be weighed against the advantages and might preclude the use of some blocks where the risk of intravascular needle placement is high, e.g. axillary or subclavian brachial plexus, median nerve at the elbow, retrobulbar and popliteal blocks.

Pneumothorax

The supraclavicular approaches to the brachial plexus, intercostal nerve, interpleural and thoracic paravertebral blocks have the potential to produce a pneumothorax. The published figures for the incidence following brachial plexus blocks vary according to the use of confirmatory X-rays (complicated by the arbitrary assessment of volume and therefore clinical importance) but may be up to 6%. The sudden onset of pleuritic pain, dyspnoea or a dry cough may be the first sign of a pneumothorax which must be confirmed by chest X-ray, although pneumothorax may not present clinically for up to 24 hours after the technique was performed. If the volume is significant (over 20% of the hemithorax) or if general anaesthesia with nitrous oxide is required, the pneumothorax must be drained. Usually pneumothoraces will resolve with conservative management and careful observation.

Widespread block

Peripheral blocks which are performed adjacent to the central neuraxis (such as brachial plexus and paravertebral blocks) have the potential to spread centrally thus producing bilateral effects. This may occur because of epidural block in the case of paravertebral blocks or by spread beneath the deep cervical fascia in the case of interscalene brachial plexus blocks. Brachial plexus blockade may also cause stellate ganglion blockade, inducing Horner's syndrome and phrenic nerve blockade which may result in dyspnoea.

Complications of patient management

Pre-existing neural pathology

Patients with pre-existing peripheral neuropathy due to diabetes mellitus, multiple sclerosis or other neurological diseases, require special consideration because any post-operative deterioration in their neurological status will undoubtedly be attributed to the nerve block, despite evidence in the literature that changes in the patients' symptoms are not commonly due to the technique itself. If there is clear clinical benefit to be gained from using a regional technique, pre-existing nerve lesions should be carefully documented pre-operatively and the patient should be thoroughly informed of the risks and benefits of the technique which should be performed by an experienced practitioner of regional anaesthesia.

Inappropriate sedation

The decision about whether to sedate or anaesthetise a patient as part of the peri-operative management must be addressed carefully during the pre-operative visit. It can be as difficult to manage an over-sedated patient as it is to cope with an uncooperative patient frightened by the whole process of local anaesthesia and surgery and whose anxiety can manifest itself in autonomic overactivity or acute psychological distress. Both these scenarios can result in a crisis of patient management requiring rapid induction of general anaesthesia to regain control of the situation. A patient may become disturbed during a previously well managed procedure if the surgeon strays out of the anaesthetised territory either directly by incising unblocked territory or indirectly by putting traction on un-anaesthetised structures within the blocked area. Such a situation is best avoided by adapting the surgical technique and by prior discussion of the surgical needs.

Vasovagal faint

This common complication of regional anaesthesia can have serious consequences if not handled quickly and correctly. It may be volunteered by patients as evidence of a previous 'allergy' to local anaesthetic drugs and therefore needs careful discussion with the patient. Vasovagal events may occur in people other than the patient (nurses or other observers) when the technique is being performed thus presenting the anaesthetist with two patients, one of whom is now unconscious!

Faulty patient positioning

The manner in which the patient is positioned after the establishment of the block is important for two main reasons. First, the anaesthetised portion of the body needs protection from pressure, high temperature and other potentially damaging forces as the patient will be unable to protect that part of their body in the normal way. Similarly, hyperextension or flexion of anaesthetised joints must be avoided to prevent neural or cutaneous damage. Secondly, if the conscious patient is to undergo surgery lasting more than 30 minutes, then they must be made as comfortable as possible to avoid increasing discomfort and consequent fidgeting and non-cooperation.

Tourniquet pressure

Pneumatic or elastic tourniquets are frequently used for limb or digit surgery and are associated with a risk of peripheral nerve and muscle damage if applied for an undue length of time or with excessive pressure over a small surface area. Careful control of total tourniquet time, padding of the cuff (which must be of the correct size) and appropriate inflation pressure will minimise such complications. If used in conjunction with peripheral nerve blockade, the tourniquet may cause patient discomfort when inflated on an unblocked part of the limb for more than a few minutes. The use of elastic tourniquets around the base of digits, particularly when combined with digital nerve blocks, can cause damage to the digital nerves and should be discouraged.

Compartment syndrome

Increased pressure in the myofascial compartments of a traumatised limb, due to oedema or haematoma, can cause neural damage from prolonged ischaemia. Pain on passive movement of the affected limb, tense swelling and decreased peripheral pulses are the cardinal signs. Urgent fasciotomy and excision of damaged tissue to prevent permanent nerve damage may be required. Many trauma patients are denied the benefits of a nerve block because of concerns that the block will mask the pain and thus delay diagnosis. If a patient is to undergo surgery to a limb which will decompress the affected compartments, then regional anaesthesia is not contraindicated and may well increase perfusion of the affected area. If there is concern about compartment syndrome occurring at a later stage, then intracompartmental pressure monitoring should be instituted as a more sensitive monitor than the onset of pain. Careful post-operative monitoring of circulation and skin colour plus 'breakthrough pain' is still necessary and full consultation with surgical colleagues should enable proper analgesia to be established without unnecessary risk.

Drug related complications

Local anaesthetic drugs have very powerful membrane stabilising properties and require careful use if serious toxicity is to be avoided. Unfortunately, partly because of the way in which they are traditionally labelled by percentage rather than in mg/ml concentration, many users are unaware of the concept of a safe dose (either in volume or drug mass) and inject potentially lethal doses. The usually quoted maximum doses or volumes given on the drug data sheets by manufacturers are a guide but do not allow for differences in clinical use. A particular dose may be perfectly safe if injected into a relatively avascular area but may cause systemic toxicity if injected into a very vascular area, due to rapid absorption.

The clinical manifestations of toxicity feature initial central nervous excitation at low plasma levels, followed by generalised CNS depression if the plasma levels rise sufficiently high (Fig. 1.3).

FACTORS INFLUENCING DRUG TOXICITY

- Toxicity of the drug (which is related to its anaesthetic potency)
- Pharmacokinetic properties of the local anaesthetic agent
- Rate of rise of plasma levels
- Peak plasma level
- Total fraction of unbound drug in circulation

In addition to CNS effects, local anaesthetic agents also have direct cardiovascular and peripheral vascular effects. Lidocaine is extensively used for treating cardiac dysrhythmias by decreasing the rate of depolarisation, the duration of the action potential and the refractory period. On the other hand, bupivacaine is thought to be intrinsically cardiotoxic and is associated with difficult resuscitation of ventricular dysrhythmias following the administration of a toxic dose. The particular affinity of bupivacaine for cardiac conducting tissue may dictate prolonged CPR if toxicity is severe.

Intravascular injection

Peripheral nerves are usually associated with both veins and arteries in neurovascular bundles and thus intravascular injection is a constant risk. Much of the published data on the toxic effects of intravascular injection relate to large volumes of intravenous administration

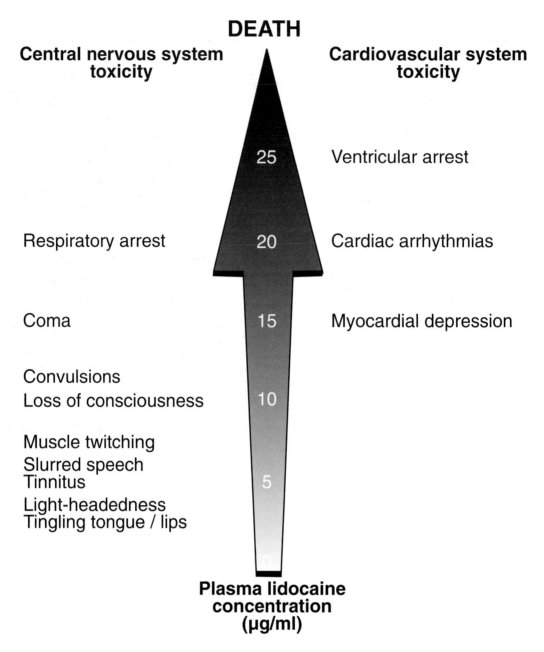

DEATH

Central nervous system toxicity

Cardiovascular system toxicity

25 — Ventricular arrest

Respiratory arrest — 20 — Cardiac arrhythmias

Coma — 15 — Myocardial depression

Convulsions
Loss of consciousness — 10

Muscle twitching
Slurred speech
Tinnitus — 5
Light-headedness
Tingling tongue / lips

Plasma lidocaine concentration (µg/ml)

Fig. 1.3
Local anaesthetic toxicity

and the correlation between venous plasma levels and the observed symptoms. Intra-arterial injection is less common but extremely dangerous. In particular, blocks performed around the head and neck carry the attendant possibility of intra-arterial injection into the carotid system, either directly or by retrograde spread, and thus even very small volumes of local anaesthetic will reach the cerebral circulation in high enough concentration to cause fatal toxicity. Similarly, injection into the vertebral artery is a particular hazard of the interscalene approach to the brachial plexus.

Drug overdose

Whereas intravascular injection will produce signs of toxicity within seconds or minutes, an overdose of local anaesthetic agent may take several hours to produce symptoms (if the rate of administration or absorption is slow) because redistribution, plasma binding and metabolism all help to reduce the plasma levels. Overdose is more usually associated with continuous administration by infusion or repeated boluses.

Anaphylactoid reactions

Patients may offer history of previous adverse reaction to local anaesthesia and say that they are 'allergic' to a particular drug. The majority of such reactions are due to intravascular injection, the effects of adrenaline in the injection or psychological reaction. The incidence of anaphylactoid and anaphylactic reactions to amide local anaesthetics is very low, with few case reports in the world literature. Some documented reactions have been shown to be due to additives such as methylparaben or metabisulphite used as preservatives. Careful history-taking will determine the precise cause of any previous adverse reaction and, if necessary, the patient should have a series of skin testing injections to confirm the reaction.

Vasoconstriction

Adrenaline (epinephrine) is the most commonly added vasoconstrictor. In dilute solution and small volume it causes few problems. The optimal dilution is 1: 200 000 with a limit of 200 µg, i.e. 40 ml with 5 µg/ml. Nevertheless, intravascular injection of only 2–3 ml of adrenaline-containing solutions or the use of large volumes, can result in systemic absorption and cause a brisk tachycardia, hypertension, palpitations and a feeling of apprehension for the patient. Adrenaline-containing solutions should not be used where the blood supply is an end artery or where the injection can cause compression of the vessels or nerve because the resultant prolonged vasoconstriction can cause tissue and neural ischaemia.

'Wrong' solutions

This complication is one of bad management. If the technique is correctly carried out and all solutions are checked properly, then only a labelled syringe of local anaesthetic agent should be available for injection.

Methaemoglobinaemia

Methaemoglobinaemia is a specific side effect of the absorption of a large dose (approximately 600 mg) of prilocaine. Cyanosis may be seen and this is due to the degradation of prilocaine into o-toluidine in the liver with the subsequent oxidation of haemoglobin to methaemoglobin. It is not clinically significant, and reverts spontaneously, unless the patient has disordered oxygen-carrying capacity. Alternatively, cyanosis may be reversed with an intravenous injection of methylene blue (1 mg/kg).

Management of complications

Most complications can be prevented by attention to detail in assessing the patient, planning and performing the block, and in monitoring the patient closely during and after the operation.

Minor adverse effects (light-headedness, circumoral tingling) need no special treatment beyond stopping the injection. Management of other adverse effects is shown in Table 1.6. First-line management of minor complications should follow a protocol, for example, administer supplementary oxygen, monitor cardiovascular function and maintain verbal contact with the patient.

Table 1.6 Management of adverse effects of regional anaesthesia

Adverse effect	Presentation	Management
psychological	distress	reassurance supplementary oxygen
	vasovagal syncope with bradycardia/hypotension	atropine 600 µg or glycopyrrolate 300 µg i.v. fluids i.v. consider ephedrine 3 mg increments i.v.
anaphylactoid reactions		supplementary oxygen intravenous colloid consider i.v. steroids/antihistamines
anaphylactic reaction		intubation, ventilation with oxygen intravenous colloid adrenaline 0.5 ml of 1: 1000 initial dose i.v. steroids (hydrocortisone 100–300 mg i.v.) antihistamine (chlorpheniramine 10–20 mg i.v.)
central nervous toxicity	mild	supplementary oxygen reassurance
	severe	intubation, ventilation with oxygen anticonvulsants (diazepam/thiopentone increments) circulatory support
cardiovascular depression	mild	supplementary oxygen elevate legs intravenous crystalloid
	severe	bradycardia – atropine 600 µg i.v. hypotension – ephedrine 3 mg increments i.v. cardiopulmonary resuscitation as indicated by the relevant international body (for example European Resuscitation Council)

Operative site

Foot and ankle

Introduction

The nerves supplying the foot are easy to locate and can be blocked with a high degree of success. Contrary to existing texts, there is no need for the prone position and thus little inconvenience for either patient or anaesthetist. Ankle block does not deserve its reputation as 'difficult and unpredictable'.

The nerve supply to the foot is comprised of five terminal nerves: superficial and deep peroneal, saphenous, sural and tibial. It is rarely necessary to block more than two or three nerves in combination unless the surgery is very extensive in which case a more proximal approach such as the popliteal block (pp. 72–73) or sciatic nerve block (pp. 78–86) will be more appropriate.

Dorsum of the foot

The skin and deeper structures of the dorsum of the foot are supplied by the superficial and deep peroneal nerves, which are the terminal branches of the common peroneal nerve (L4, 5–S 1, 2).

Deep peroneal nerve

The deep peroneal nerve innervates muscle and bone underlying the dorsum and the metatarso–phalangeal joints of the second, third and fourth toes. Cutaneous innervation is limited to the adjacent sides of the great and second toes (Fig. 2.1.1).

Superficial peroneal nerve

The superficial peroneal nerve innervates the skin of the dorsum of the foot, the medial side of the great toe and the dorsal surface of all the toes, except those areas innervated by the deep peroneal nerve (Fig. 2.1.2). The lateral aspect of the 5th toe is supplied by the sural nerve.

Applied anatomy

Superficial and deep peroneal nerves are invariably blocked in combination because of the overlapping cutaneous territories. One point of needle insertion may be used for both techniques.

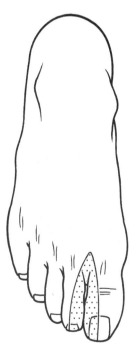

Fig. 2.1.1
Cutaneous innervation of the deep peroneal nerve

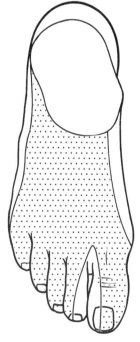

Fig. 2.1.2
Cutaneous innervation of the superficial peroneal nerve

Medial surface of the foot

Saphenous nerve

The saphenous nerve (L2, 3, 4) divides into two branches at the level of the medial malleolus, one branch innervates the skin overlying the ankle and the other continues forward to supply the medial aspect of the foot as far distal as the metatarso–phalangeal joint of the great toe, although the combined territory is variable (Fig. 2.1.3).

Applied anatomy

Although the saphenous nerve can be blocked at the ankle, it may be more appropriate to use a more proximal technique, for example at the level of the tibial plateau. This is especially suitable if the proposed operation site lies around the medial malleolus. In both approaches the nerve is easily blocked by subcutaneous infiltration.

Sole of the foot

The skin and superficial tissues of the sole of the foot are supplied by four branches of the tibial nerve, L4, 5–S1, 2, 3 (Fig. 2.1.4).

Medial calcaneal nerve

The medial calcaneal nerve branches off the tibial nerve behind the medial malleolus and pierces the flexor retinaculum to innervate the skin of the heel and the postero-medial surface of the sole. The tibial nerve divides at the level of the medial malleolus into the medial and lateral plantar nerves underneath the flexor retinaculum.

Medial plantar nerve

The medial plantar nerve innervates the antero-medial surface of the sole and the plantar surface of the medial three and a half toes.

Lateral plantar nerve

The lateral plantar nerve innervates the antero-lateral surface of the sole and the plantar surface of the lateral one and a half toes.

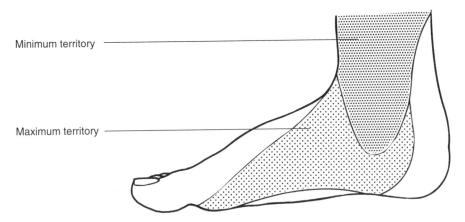

Minimum territory

Maximum territory

Fig. 2.1.3
Cutaneous innervation of the saphenous nerve

Sural nerve

The sural nerve branches off the tibial nerve in the popliteal fossa. It runs between the lateral malleolus and the calcaneum to innervate the lateral border of the foot and little toe.

Applied anatomy

The medial calcaneal and the medial and lateral plantar nerves all pass deep to the flexor retinaculum and thus may all be blocked by a single injection beneath the retinaculum at a point midway between the heel and the sustentaculum tali, which can be palpated as a bony ridge just below the medial malleolus. In most cases all three branches will be blocked equally but it is possible for one or more of the nerves to be partially blocked, especially if too small a volume of local anaesthetic is used.

The cutaneous territories of each nerve have a varied distribution and do not always correspond with the underlying deeper structures. Therefore, it is always advisable to block adjacent nerves especially if the site of surgery is close to the boundary of a nerve territory. Thus, the sural, the superficial and deep peroneal nerves may need to be blocked to ensure complete anaesthesia at the boundaries of the sole of the foot.

Toes

Digital nerves

The toes are each innervated by four digital nerves, two dorsal and two ventral. The digital nerves are the terminal branches of the peroneal nerves (dorsally) and the tibial nerve (ventrally). They are formed at the level of the bases of the metatarsals from where they pass distally in close approximation to the bones of each digit.

Applied anatomy

In the event that more proximal blocks of the foot have not been adequate in providing analgesia of the affected digit, the appropriate digital nerves can be blocked to reinforce the analgesia.

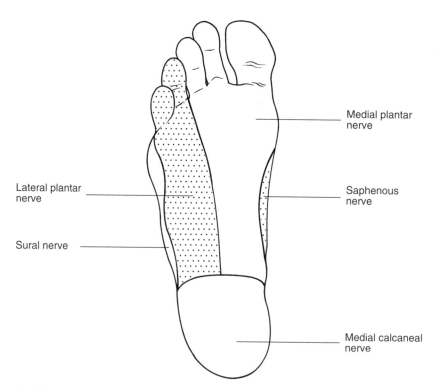

Fig. 2.1.4
Cutaneous innervation of the sole of the foot

INDICATIONS

- Minor foot surgery – Nerve blocks at the ankle or of the digital nerves are suitable for a variety of minor operations and for the debridement and suturing of lacerations.
- Complex foot surgery – The sciatic nerve can be blocked in the popliteal fossa and combined if necessary with a saphenous nerve block to provide complete anaesthesia of the lower leg and foot. Alternatively, nerve blockade at the ankle will restrict motor and sensory block to the foot, leaving the extensor and flexor muscles of the lower leg unaffected. This can be of advantage in some forms of foot surgery and allows the patient early post-operative control of the leg whilst maintaining analgesia of the foot.

Lower limb

Introduction

Commonly, when regional anaesthesia is employed during lower limb surgery, practitioners limit their techniques to spinal and epidural approaches without considering the advantages that long-lasting discrete nerve blockade offers for intra- and post-operative analgesia. Difficulty with locating deep nerves, the need to combine two or more nerve blocks and lack of experience with a PNS all contribute to this decision. For those who are prepared to

learn the necessary skills for peripheral nerve blocks in the lower limb, the benefits of up to 36 hours high quality analgesia can be achieved without the disadvantages of bladder and bowel disturbance and the bilateral immobility associated with central blockade.

The nerve supply to the lower limb is comprised of two plexuses (lumbar and sacral) and five major terminal nerves (femoral, obturator, lateral cutaneous, sciatic and posterior cutaneous nerve of thigh).

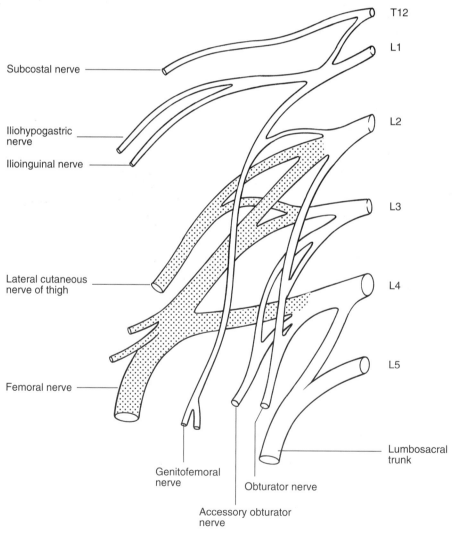

Fig. 2.2.1
Lumbar plexus

Lumbar plexus

The lumbar plexus is formed from the anterior divisions of L1 to L4 (Fig. 2.2.1) which combine in a series of loops within the substance of the psoas major muscle, just in front of the transverse processes of the lumbar vertebrae. Six main terminal nerves arise from these loops. The three proximal ones, the iliohypogastric, the ilioinguinal (T12–L1) and the genitofemoral (L1, 2) supply muscular and cutaneous branches to the lower abdomen and the more proximal part of the lower limb. The three distal nerves, the femoral nerve (L2, 3, 4), the lateral cutaneous nerve of thigh (L2, 3) and the obturator nerve (L2, 3, 4) leave the plexus to innervate the majority of cutaneous and deeper structures above the knee whilst the largest cutaneous branch of the femoral nerve, the saphenous nerve, supplies cutaneous innervation below the knee.

Femoral nerve

The femoral nerve is the largest branch of the plexus. It enters the leg by passing deep to the inguinal ligament immediately lateral to the femoral vessels. The nerve is invested in its own fascial sheath within the iliopectineal fascia running deep to the fascia lata. It immediately divides into an anterior and posterior division. The anterior division supplies one muscle – the sartorious – and two cutaneous nerves which innervate the anterior and medial aspects of the thigh, including the skin overlying the knee. The posterior division supplies motor fibres to the quadriceps femoris, articular fibres to the knee joint and ends as the saphenous nerve (q.v.).

Obturator nerve

The obturator nerve enters the leg through the upper part of the obturator foramen, where it divides into a posterior and anterior branch which are separated by the adductor brevis muscle. Both branches have motor and sensory fibres. The anterior branch supplies sensory fibres to the hip and the medial aspect of the thigh and also sends fibres to the subsartorial plexus with the femoral nerve. The posterior branch sends fibres to the capsule of the knee.

Lateral cutaneous nerve of thigh

The lateral cutaneous nerve of thigh (LCNT) is sensory only and innervates a variable area of skin on the lateral aspect of the thigh as far distal as the patella (Fig. 2.2.2).

Applied anatomy

The lumbar plexus can be blocked by two proximal techniques; the lumbar paravertebral approach, which blocks the nerve roots, and the lumbar plexus block (sometimes called the psoas compartment block) which blocks the loops of the plexus. However, the plexus can also be approached by a distal technique popularised by A. D. Winnie and known as the inguinal paravascular or '3 in 1' block (pp. 76–77).

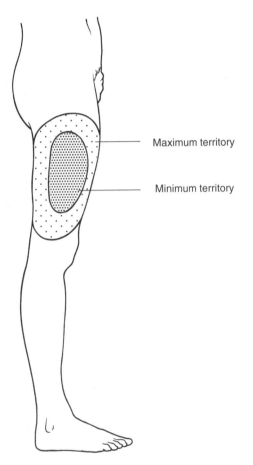

Maximum territory

Minimum territory

Fig. 2.2.2
Cutaneous innervation of the lateral cutaneous nerve of thigh

Sacral plexus

The sacral plexus (Fig. 2.2.3) is formed from the lumbosacral trunk (the ventral rami of L4–5 and the ventral rami of S1, 2 and 3). The plexus lies on the piriformis muscle over the anterior surface of the sacrum and gives rise to several nerves within the pelvis but only two terminal nerves to the leg, the sciatic nerve and the posterior cutaneous nerve of thigh which both leave the pelvis through the greater sciatic foramen and are in close proximity as they descend down the back of the thigh.

Sciatic nerve

The sciatic nerve (L4, 5, S1, 2, 3) is the largest nerve in the body with a maximum width of 2 cm as it exits the pelvis. The point of division into two components (peroneal and tibial nerves) is variable, occurring anywhere from the sciatic foramen to the lower part of the thigh. In the thigh, the sciatic nerve gives off articular branches to the hip joint and motor branches to the hamstring muscles. The tibial nerve, which is the larger of the two branches, supplies articular branches to the knee and

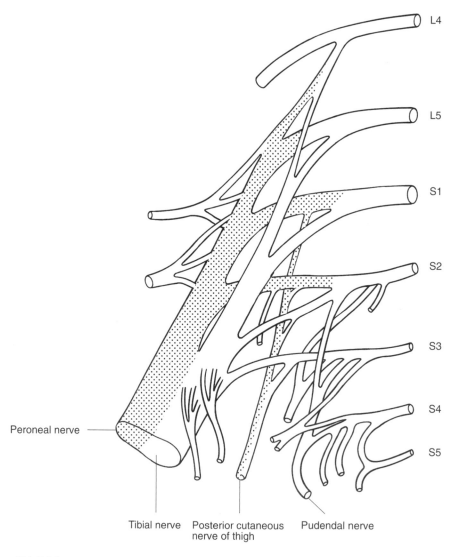

Peroneal nerve

Tibial nerve

Posterior cutaneous nerve of thigh

Pudendal nerve

L4

L5

S1

S2

S3

S4

S5

Fig. 2.2.3
Sacral plexus

ankle joints, muscular branches to the calf muscles and the plantar muscles of the foot. In the popliteal fossa, the tibial nerve gives origin to the sural nerve which innervates the postero-lateral skin of the lower leg (Fig. 2.2.4). The peroneal nerve supplies cutaneous innervation to the proximal, lateral part of the lower leg as well as the dorsum of the foot and articular branches to the knee.

Posterior cutaneous nerve of the thigh

The posterior cutaneous nerve of the thigh (S1, 2, 3) innervates the posterior aspect of the thigh and upper part of the calf.

Applied anatomy

Because the posterior cutaneous nerve of thigh is so closely associated with the sciatic nerve as they exit the greater sciatic foramen, for all practical purposes, the two nerves are blocked together when sciatic blockade (pp. 78–86) is used.

The sacral plexus lies immediately anterior to the sacrum and can only be approached via the trans-sacral canals on the posterior surface. This requires four separate injections, each of which carries significant risk of damage to the nerves and the deeper pelvic structures. As a caudal injection is technically easier and can achieve the same effect, it should be used in preference to a sacral plexus block.

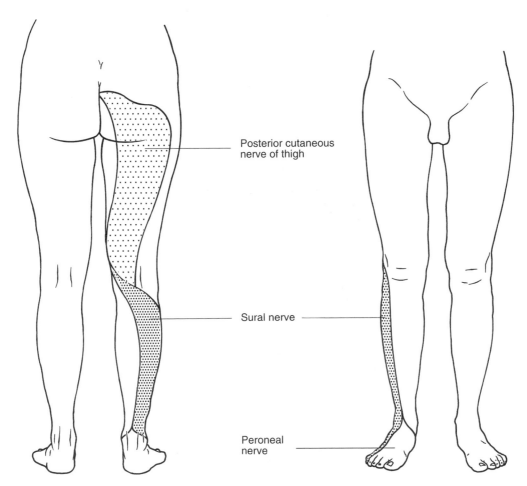

Posterior cutaneous nerve of thigh

Sural nerve

Peroneal nerve

Fig. 2.2.4
Cutaneous innervation of the sciatic nerve

The way in which the territories of the five nerves innervating the lower limb overlap generally results in multiple nerve blocks being necessary to achieve adequate surgical anaesthesia over a particular field. Most commonly, the sciatic nerve and the femoral nerve are both blocked to ensure adequate anaesthesia of the lower limb although the obturator and the LCNT may also require blockade.

INDICATIONS

- Hip joint surgery – This can be effectively undertaken if a paravertebral or lumbar plexus block is used where, for instance, a spinal or epidural technique is contra-indicated. A '3 in 1' block is not so effective for this purpose because it does not so reliably block the LCNT and would not be expected to block the iliohypogastric and ilioinguinal nerves which innervate the skin overlying the iliac crest and buttock. For complete anaesthesia of the hip joint, a sciatic nerve block is needed in combination with the plexus block. Peripheral nerve blocks, combined with light general anaesthesia may prove especially useful in the frail elderly patient. Femoral, LCNT, sciatic and iliac crest blocks will be needed in combination. Pay careful attention to volume and the total dose of local anaesthetic agent.
- Knee joint surgery – A '3 in 1' block plus a sciatic nerve block provides profound intra-operative and post-operative analgesia for all types of knee surgery. It is important to remember that Hilton's law applies. In respect of the knee joint, the femoral, sciatic, LCNT and obturator all supply fibres to the joint, either directly or via neural plexuses within the thigh. Thus it may be preferable to consider discrete nerve block of each individual nerve, rather than rely on a plexus block.
- Long bone surgery – Femoral nerve and sciatic nerve blocks in combination can be used for surgery to both the femur and the tibia and fibula.
- Ankle joint surgery – A popliteal nerve block and a saphenous nerve block at the knee are the best combination.
- Trauma – Femoral nerve blocks are very helpful in the management of pain following bony or soft tissue injury of the thigh, both in adults and children. Below the knee, sciatic and femoral blocks are equally useful although it is important to consider the risk of compartment syndrome developing and its symptoms being masked. This also applies to injuries of the lower part of the arm where there are also interosseous compartments.
- Sympathetic blockade – Although the lumbar sympathetic chain is separate from the somatic nerve supply, there is considerable interconnection with somatic nerves. Thus, if the major nerves of the leg are blocked then significant sympathetic nerve blockade results offering clinically useful vasodilatation for patients with peripheral vascular disease, especially in the management of ischaemic rest pain and pre-gangrenous changes. The role of nerve sheath catheters in improving local circulation is discussed on p. 164.

Abdomen and thorax

Introduction

For the majority of operations within the abdomen, the regional anaesthetic technique of choice is central neural blockade using a lumbar epidural or spinal which are effective against both somatic and visceral pain. The autonomic nerve blockade offers important benefits by preserving gut function, maintaining blood flow and modifying the neuro-humoral responses to surgical stress.

It is important to remember that within the abdomen, all painful stimuli arising from the visceral organs (including the peritoneum) are relayed via sympathetic visceral nociceptor nerve fibres to the spinal cord. Peripheral nerve blockade will not affect viscerally mediated pain – if bowel is manipulated during herniorrhaphy, for example. Nevertheless, for operations which require mainly somatic analgesia or where bilateral analgesia is inappropriate and unnecessary, peripheral nerve blocks are very effective at providing high quality post-operative analgesia.

Abdominal wall

Spinal nerves

The anterior abdominal wall is innervated by the 7th to the 12th thoracic nerves except in the inguinal area where the iliohypogastric and ilioinguinal nerves contribute to the somatic nerve supply. The nerves enter the abdominal wall through the transversus abdominis muscle and innervate the external and internal oblique muscles and the overlying skin before entering the posterior aspect of the rectus sheath. Here the nerves supply separate sections of the rectus muscles before leaving the anterior aspect of the sheath to innervate the midline skin of the abdomen. The subcostal nerve (T12) sends fibres to the 1st lumbar nerve and its lateral cutaneous branch runs over the iliac crest to innervate the skin of the lateral aspect of the buttock as far as the greater trochanter.

Lumbar plexus

The majority of the lumbar plexus neurones innervate the lower limb. The nerve roots of L1 and L2, however, together with fibres from T12 supply the lowest cutaneous innervation of the abdominal wall, the suprapubic area and parts of the external genitalia. The fibres of T12 combine with L1 to form the iliohypogastric and ilioinguinal nerves (Fig. 2.3.1) which sweep around the medial surface of the iliac crest and at a point 1–2 cm medial to the anterior superior iliac spine (ASIS) they are separated by the internal oblique muscle. The iliohypogastric nerve and the subcostal nerves lie between the internal oblique muscle and the aponeurosis of the external oblique while the ilioinguinal nerve lies deep to the internal oblique muscle. The iliohypogastric nerve innervates the skin overlying the lateral aspect of the buttock and then runs medially and superficial to the inguinal canal, to innervate the skin over the pubis. The ilioinguinal nerve enters the inguinal canal, accompanies the spermatic cord and supplies the skin of the root of the penis and anterior part of the scrotum (male) and the mons pubis and labia majora (female). In addition, the ilioinguinal nerve innervates the skin of the upper and inner aspect of the thigh (Fig. 2.3.1). The genitofemoral nerve (L1, 2) has two branches. The genital branch enters the inguinal canal and supplies the spermatic cord and innervates the same cutaneous area as the ilioinguinal nerve. The femoral branch innervates the skin overlying the femoral triangle.

Pudendal nerve

The pudendal nerve (S2, 3, 4) arises from the sacral plexus and gives rise to the dorsal nerve of penis (clitoris) and the perineal nerve. Each dorsal nerve passes under the pubic symphysis accompanied by the dorsal artery and vein running beneath the deep fascia of the penis into the glans penis to supply the shaft and glans of the penis. The ventral surface and root of the penis are innervated by branches of the perineal nerve. The perineal nerve also innervates the infero-posterior aspects of the scrotum, and the labia majora in the female (Figs. 2.3.2, 2.3.3).

Applied anatomy

Peripheral nerve block of the abdominal wall will only anaesthetise the somatic nerve supply to the abdomen. Such techniques are thus only

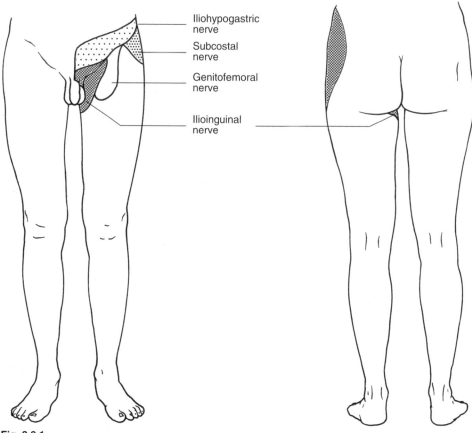

Fig. 2.3.1
Cutaneous innervation of the iliohypogastric and ilioinguinal nerves

Iliohypogastric nerve

Subcostal nerve

Genitofemoral nerve

Ilioinguinal nerve

suitable for operations which do not breach the peritoneum, although if the intra-abdominal component of the procedure is limited, there may be limited visceral pain and the somatic blockade will prove sufficient. Intercostal nerve blocks (pp. 100–101) are effective for unilateral analgesia of the anterior abdominal wall. The 7–11th intercostal nerves can be blocked by the standard approach to the intercostal space but the 12th nerve can be difficult to locate under the 12th rib and therefore it is better to block this nerve more peripherally either by subcutaneous infiltration along the iliac crest (p. 93) or by performing a discrete block of the iliohypogastric nerve (pp. 96–97). Interpleural block (pp. 104–105) provides the same distribution of analgesia as intercostal blocks but its effects will extend beyond the lower thoracic dermatomes. Iliohypogastric and ilioinguinal nerve block (pp. 96–97) is particularly indicated for surgery confined to the inguinal region and can be usefully combined with genitofemoral nerve block. This combination of

nerve blocks is called the inguinal field block to denote the area of analgesia produced.

INDICATIONS

- Abdominal surgery – Intercostal blocks are well established in the management of post-operative pain from cholecystectomy. Recently, interpleural analgesia has been increasingly used for both laparoscopic and open cholecystectomy and nephrectomy. Rectus sheath blocks will abolish pain from midline or paramedian incisions and are useful for secondary closure of wounds, colostomies, umbilical hernias and other abdominal wall operations.
- Inguinal herniorrhaphy – The inguinal field block is suitable in both conscious and anaesthetised patients for hernia surgery and is especially useful in day surgery as it allows light general anaesthesia to be used,

thus allowing a more rapid return to 'street fitness' as well as offering prolonged post-operative analgesia.

- Chronic pain conditions – Nerve entrapment syndromes occur in the abdominal wall, especially following surgery, and can be treated with appropriate intercostal nerve block(s), rectus sheath block or inguinal canal block.

External genitalia

The external genitalia have a complex cutaneous nerve supply and it is necessary to anaesthetise every nerve if complete analgesia is to be achieved. This is impractical in females and a caudal epidural injection is more sensible. In the male, the penis, the scrotum and its contents can only be anaesthetised completely if the dorsal nerve of penis, the perineal nerves, the genitofemoral and ilioinguinal nerves are all blocked.

Applied anatomy

Penile block (p. 94) requires that the pair of nerves is located immediately beneath the deep ('Buck's') fascia at the inferior surface of the pubic symphysis to ensure that the posterior branches of the nerves, which innervate the

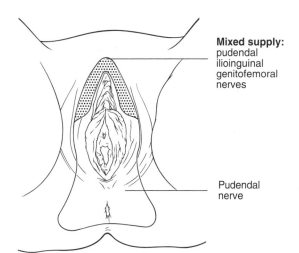

Fig. 2.3.3
Innervation of female genitalia

ventral surface, are affected, otherwise analgesia may be incomplete. Inguinal canal block (pp. 96–97) will block the ilioinguinal and genitofemoral nerves as well as the spermatic cord and the testicle and is, therefore, an essential technique to learn for testicular and scrotal surgery. Scrotal infiltration (p. 95) along the line of anticipated incision is the most practical method of blocking the fibres of the perineal nerve which supply the scrotum.

INDICATIONS

- Penile surgery – Penile blocks compare equally well with caudal blocks for circumcision and other penile surgery and avoid the inevitable side effects of caudals – bladder and bowel dysfunction and motor dysfunction in the legs. Depending on the type and site of surgery, a penile block may need to be combined with other blocks.
- Scrotal/testicular surgery – Peripheral nerve blockade for testicular and scrotal surgery can be as effective as caudal or epidural approaches. With respect to the inguinal approach to orchidopexy, an inguinal field block is the technique of choice but where testicular surgery is confined to the scrotum, an inguinal canal block with scrotal infiltration will be sufficient.

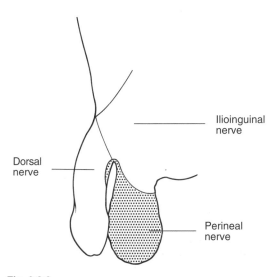

Fig. 2.3.2
Innervation of male genitalia

Thorax

For the majority of operations within the chest the regional anaesthetic technique of choice is central neural blockade using a thoracic epidural. Epidural analgesia is effective against both somatic and visceral pain and the autonomic nerve blockade offers important benefits by maintaining blood flow and modifying the neuro-humoral responses to surgical stress.

It is important to remember that within the cavities of the chest all painful stimuli arising from the visceral organs (including the pleura) are relayed via sympathetic visceral nociceptor nerve fibres to the spinal cord; *thus, peripheral nerve blockade will not affect viscerally mediated pain*. Nevertheless, for operations which require mainly somatic analgesia or where bilateral analgesia is inappropriate and unnecessary, peripheral nerve blocks are very effective at providing high quality post-operative analgesia.

Spinal nerves

The spinal cord gives rise to twelve pairs of thoracic nerves (T1–T12) which share a number of common characteristics. All contain mixed motor, sensory and autonomic fibres and within the paravertebral space, divide into a small dorsal and larger ventral nerve. The dorsal nerves supply the erector spinae muscles and sensory fibres to the skin and deep structures of the posterior aspect of the trunk. The ventral nerves supply the lateral and anterior parts of the trunk and each is contained within the neurovascular bundle of the intercostal space beneath the inferior aspect of the rib. Each nerve gives rise to a lateral branch and then continues forward to innervate the anterior aspect of the trunk. The sensory limits of each nerve are conventionally depicted as dermatomes on the skin surface (Fig. 2.3.4), although there is considerable overlap between the individual dermatomes. T5, T7, T10 and T12 represent important landmarks on the trunk for the assessment of the spread of epidural or spinal analgesia.

As a result of the downward and forward path of the thoracic nerves, posterior innervation stops at the level of the 12th thoracic spine. Anteriorly, however, the thoracic nerves supply the anterior abdominal wall and the subcostal nerve (T12) sends fibres to the 1st lumbar nerve and its lateral cutaneous branch runs over the iliac crest to innervate the skin of the lateral aspect of the buttock as far as the greater trochanter.

Chest wall

The number of nerves to be blocked will depend on the size and location of the injury or incision. It is necessary to block one nerve proximal and one distal to the selected nerve(s) because of the overlap of dermatomes. For example, a Kocher's subcostal incision in the T7–8 dermatomes also requires T6 and T9 to be blocked for complete coverage.

Applied anatomy

For analgesia of the posterior part of the chest wall, a thoracic paravertebral injection (pp. 102–103), preferably with catheter insertion is more suitable than intercostal nerve injections because the dorsal nerve is more reliably blocked and as the spread of a paravertebral injection is greater, fewer injections are required. Intercostal nerve blocks provide effective analgesia in the lateral and anterior parts of the chest wall. The technique is relatively easy to perform on the 6–11th nerves as these ribs are easy to palpate but the scapula can obscure the higher ribs, thus the approach needs to be made more anteriorly which can reduce the effectiveness. Interpleural block (pp. 104–105) is thought to achieve its effects by diffusion of local anaesthetic agent through the parietal layer of pleura causing blockade of the intercostal nerves, the sympathetic chain (and possibly the phrenic nerve). The block is not segmental and there may be little evidence of sensory anaesthesia. The spread of solution is greatly affected by gravity and the patient can thus be positioned so as to maximise the spread to the desired part of the pleural space. Tipping the patient head down in the supine position will block the upper thoracic nerves and the sympathetic chain and can induce Horner's syndrome.

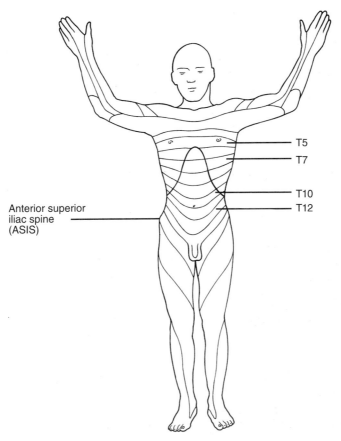

Anterior superior
iliac spine
(ASIS)

T5
T7
T10
T12

Fig. 2.3.4
Dermatomes of the abdomen and thorax

INDICATIONS

- Chest wall trauma – Fractured ribs can be treated by single injections around the appropriate intercostal nerves which may need to be repeated every 6–8 hours. Alternatively catheters may be inserted into the intercostal spaces and a constant infusion of local anaesthetic solution or repeated bolus injections administered. Where there are multiple unilateral fractures, a paravertebral catheter is more appropriate because of the greater spread of solution. Thus, a larger area of analgesia can be obtained from one catheter insertion and smaller volumes of local anaesthetic can be used. Alternatively, if the patient requires chest drains to be inserted, these can be used to effect interpleural analgesia.

- Chest wall surgery – Interpleural blocks provide good analgesia for mastectomy or other breast operations. For thoracotomy incisions, a thoracic paravertebral injection offers better analgesia than intercostal blocks and because the chest is open, the surgeon can supervise the insertion of the catheter under direct vision.
- Chronic pain conditions – Nerve entrapment syndromes, thoracic spine pain and intercostal neuralgia may respond to paravertebral or intercostal blockade.
- Bilateral or midline surgery or trauma – There is no place for bilateral intercostal, interpleural or paravertebral blocks because of the associated risks of drug toxicity and the need for multiple injection sites. A thoracic epidural is the technique of choice.

Upper limb

Introduction

With the exception of the cutaneous supply to the upper, medial aspect of the arm and the uppermost aspect of the shoulder, the arm receives its entire nerve supply from the brachial plexus. Thus, the potential exists to provide peri-operative anaesthesia and prolonged post-operative analgesia from a single injection into the brachial plexus. In practice, the majority of operations on the upper limb are carried out distal to the elbow and this allows for the use of individual nerve blocks, either singly or in combination, to limit motor and sensory deficit to the nerve territories of the operative site. The combination of a short duration brachial plexus block and long-lasting peripheral nerve blocks may be the ideal. This combination allows early recovery of the shoulder and upper arm, which is important for early mobilisation and limb protection, while maintaining good peripheral analgesia.

Brachial plexus

The structure of the plexus is complex by virtue of the repeated combination and division of its original five roots. The plexus gives rise to a total of 21 nerves (Fig. 2.4.1). Of the nine nerves which arise above the clavicle, the suprascapular is the only sensory nerve and is the only one which can be blocked as a discrete technique. The major terminal nerves to the upper limb arising below the clavicle are shown in Table 2.1.

Note. The medial cutaneous nerves of arm and forearm arise directly from the medial cord of the brachial plexus.

The neuro-anatomical configuration of the brachial plexus may be simplified by referring to Table 2.2 and Figure 2.4.1 which demonstrate the major structural components and their relationships.

Applied anatomy

The most relevant structure, in terms of ensuring the success of a brachial plexus block, is the fascial sheath which invests the whole of the plexus from the scalene muscles down to the midpoint of the upper arm. Between these two points, the level of entry into the fascia will greatly influence which components are preferentially blocked, and thus the resulting pattern of block, but the volume injected also has a major effect. In general terms, with the interscalene approach to the brachial plexus, made at the level of nerve roots, C8 and T1 are more likely to be missed because of the vertical arrangement of the roots. Thus the interscalene technique tends to fail on the ulnar side of the limb in a dermatomal distribution. In contrast, the axillary approach is made at the level of the terminal nerves and the musculocutaneous and radial nerves are the most likely nerves to be

Table 2.1 The major terminal nerves of the brachial plexus and their principle sensory branches

Nerve	Principal sensory branches
axillary	upper lateral cutaneous of arm
radial	lower lateral cutaneous of arm posterior cutaneous of arm posterior cutaneous of forearm cutaneous to dorsum of hand
ulnar	cutaneous to palm and dorsum of hand
median	cutaneous to palm and dorsum of hand
musculocutaneous	lateral cutaneous nerve of forearm

Table 2.2 The rule of '3s and 5s' applied to the structure of the brachial plexus

roots	5	C5–T1 (C4 prefixed, T2 postfixed)
trunks	3	superior (C5–6) middle (C7) inferior (C8–T1)
divisions	3 3	anterior posterior
cords	3	lateral medial posterior
terminal nerves	5	median (lateral, medial cords) musculocutaneous (lateral cord) ulnar (medial cord) axillary (posterior cord) radial (posterior cord)

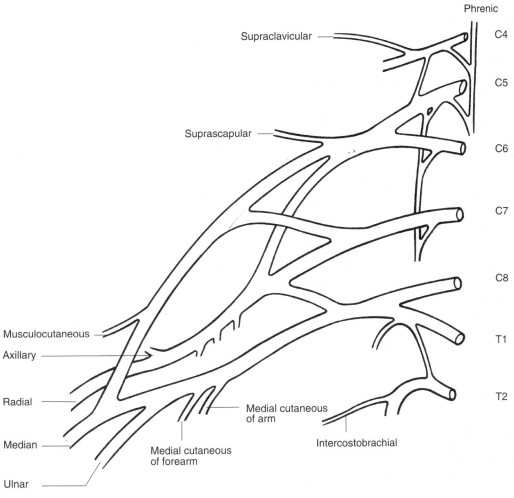

Fig. 2.4.1
Brachial plexus

inadequately blocked resulting in failure within a terminal nerve distribution. With the supraclavicular approach, injection is made at the level of the trunks. As there are only three components at this level, the failure rate should be low but if it does occur, it will be in a mixed distribution of terminal nerve and dermatomes derived from the inferior trunk.

The choice of approach depends primarily on the proposed site of surgery because the success rates of the three approaches vary. In general terms, the interscalene approach is best for proximal surgery (including the shoulder), the supraclavicular approach for the upper arm, elbow and radial side of forearm, and the axillary approach for the hand, wrist and ulnar side of forearm. However, to become proficient

at all three approaches requires considerable experience and for general use, the supraclavicular approach can be modified to offer the best results by adjusting the volume of local anaesthetic used and by using digital pressure to encourage spread proximally or distally as necessary.

Peripheral nerves

All the motor and sensory nerves to the upper limb derive from the infraclavicular part of the brachial plexus. The interconnection of the original five cervical nerve roots means that the cutaneous distribution of the individual nerve territories differs from the dermatomal pattern (Figs 2.4.2, 2.4.3) and that the muscular and other deep structures supplied by a nerve do not underlie the sensory distribution of that nerve. Thus blockade of the ulnar nerve at the elbow will produce sensory loss on the ulnar side of the hand but motor loss in the flexor muscles of the forearm. These points are important when planning suitable techniques. It is usually necessary to block adjoining nerve territories for the majority of operations because there is considerable overlap and variation in the distribution of the peripheral nerves.

Five terminal nerves to the lower arm and hand (ulnar, radial, median, lateral cutaneous and medial cutaneous nerves of forearm) can be blocked at the elbow (pp. 118–125) and the ulnar, median and radial nerves can also be blocked at the wrist (pp. 126–133). The posterior cutaneous nerve of forearm cannot be blocked discretely at the elbow; this must either be done in

conjunction with a brachial plexus block or by local infiltration (pp. 124–125).

The cutaneous innervation of the upper arm (medial, lateral and posterior cutaneous nerves of arm and the axillary nerve) can only be blocked as part of a brachial plexus block and the intercostobrachial nerve has to be blocked separately in the axilla.

Elbow

Ulnar nerve

The ulnar nerve enters the forearm by passing behind the medial epicondyle of the humerus. It supplies the flexor muscles of the forearm and passes down the ulnar side of the forearm. About 5 cm above the wrist, it gives rise to the dorsal and palmar cutaneous branches and then

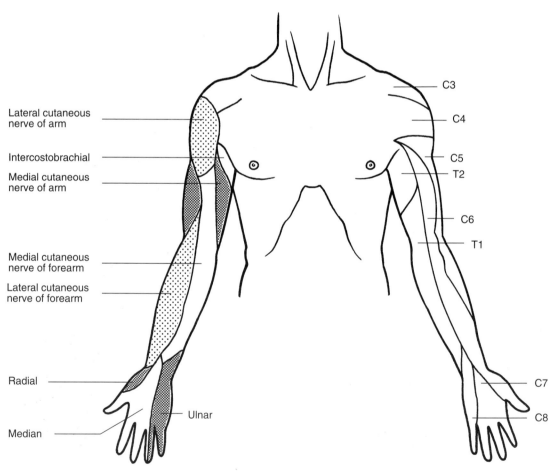

Fig. 2.4.2
Territories and dermatomes of the upper limb, anterior view

continues alongside the ulnar artery into the hand. Within the hand, it supplies some of the intrinsic muscles plus digital nerves to the little finger and the ulnar side of the ring finger. The dorsal branch innervates the dorsal aspect of the little and ring fingers and the palmar cutaneous branch supplies sensory innervation to the ulnar side of the palm.

Median nerve

The median nerve lies immediately medial to the brachial artery just proximal to the flexor skin crease of the antecubital fossa. At this point it is just deep to the bicipital aponeurosis in a groove bounded by the biceps tendon laterally and the origins of the forearm flexor muscles medially. The median nerve enters the hand deep to the flexor retinaculum in the carpal tunnel and supplies deep and superficial flexor muscles of the forearm, some of the intrinsic muscles of the hand, the skin of the palm and thenar eminence (via the palmar cutaneous branch) and digital nerves to the radial three and a half fingers.

Medial cutaneous nerve of the forearm

The medial cutaneous nerve of forearm lies subcutaneously above the bicipital aponeurosis in close relationship to the median nerve. It supplies the cutaneous innervation of the medial aspect of the forearm and some of the skin overlying the biceps in the upper arm.

Radial nerve

The radial nerve is the largest branch of the brachial plexus and supplies the extensor muscles of the upper arm and the skin overlying them before it crosses the anterior aspect of the lateral epicondyle, deep to brachioradialis

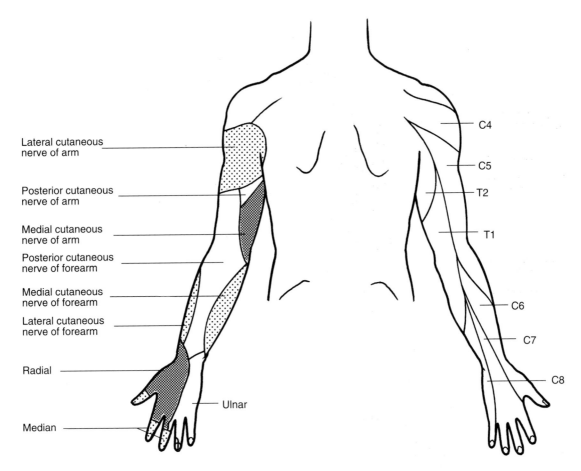

Lateral cutaneous nerve of arm

Posterior cutaneous nerve of arm

Medial cutaneous nerve of arm

Posterior cutaneous nerve of forearm

Medial cutaneous nerve of forearm

Lateral cutaneous nerve of forearm

Radial

Ulnar

Median

C4

C5

T2

T1

C6

C7

C8

Fig. 2.4.3
Territories and dermatomes of the upper limb, posterior view

muscle, and lateral to the biceps tendon in the groove between these structures to enter the forearm. Here it supplies the extensor muscles of the forearm before terminating in its cutaneous nerves to the hand.

Lateral cutaneous nerve of forearm

The lateral cutaneous nerve of forearm is the continuation of the musculocutaneous nerve and lies subcutaneously in the groove between brachioradialis and the biceps tendon and supplies the skin of the lateral aspect of the forearm.

Posterior cutaneous nerve of forearm

The posterior cutaneous nerve of forearm is a proximal branch of the radial nerve which becomes subcutaneous at the level of the elbow and descends along the postero-radial aspect of the forearm to innervate the overlying skin.

Applied anatomy

With the exception of the radial nerve, the nerves at the elbow are all very superficial. The ulnar nerve runs in a narrow sulcus behind the medial epicondyle and should not be approached within this sulcus because of the increased risk of damage either from the needle or from hydraulic pressure if excessive volume is injected into the confines of the sulcus.

INDICATIONS

- Shoulder surgery – An interscalene block is the plexus block of choice. If the incision is very proximal, separate supraclavicular nerve block may be required. For closed procedures such as arthroscopy or manipulation, a suprascapular nerve block is adequate.
- Surgery of the upper arm and elbow – A brachial plexus block is required and if the medial aspect of the arm is involved, then separate intercostobrachial nerve block may be needed as well.
- Forearm surgery – Depending on the extent and complexity of the operation, a brachial plexus block is usually the most reliable form of anaesthesia, especially if a tourniquet is required. A combination of individual nerve blocks can be used either to supplement the brachial plexus block or may be sufficient for less major surgery. Where general anaesthesia is to be given, they can be used in combination to provide good anaesthesia and post-operative analgesia.

- Trauma – Minor trauma to digits can be managed ideally with web space blocks or digital nerve blocks. If more than one digit is injured it may be more appropriate to consider discrete nerve blockade at the wrist. It is important to consider the risk of compartment syndrome occurring with closed injuries of the forearm unless the injury is to be decompressed. Brachial plexus blockade provides rapid analgesia and anaesthesia for the reduction of joint dislocations of the shoulder and elbow and for the manipulation of fractures.
- Sympathetic blockade – The brachial plexus has a rich sympathetic nerve supply which controls both arterial and venous tone. Thus brachial plexus blocks can be used for diagnostic and therapeutic management of vasospastic conditions as blood flow to compromised tissues following trauma and surgery will be maximised. The use of indwelling plexus catheters for prolonged brachial plexus analgesia is described on p. 163.

Hand and Wrist

Introduction

The hand is innervated by the terminal branches of the ulnar, median and radial nerves with some overlap at the wrist of the medial, lateral and posterior cutaneous nerves of forearm.

All five nerves can be blocked both at the elbow and the wrist and although there is considerable overlap of the adjacent nerve territories in the hand, it is rarely necessary to block more than two nerves in combination unless the surgery is very extensive. In this case it is more sensible to use a more proximal technique such as a brachial plexus block.

Wrist

Ulnar nerve

The ulnar nerve is lateral and deep to the flexor carpi ulnaris tendon, medial to the ulnar artery. The dorsal branch lies subcutaneously and dorsally at the level of the wrist joint.

Median nerve

The median nerve lies between the palmaris longus tendon medially and the flexor carpi radialis tendon laterally at a point about 2 cm proximal to the wrist. It gives rise to the palmar cutaneous branch which passes superficial to the flexor retinaculum to supply the palm and thenar eminence.

Radial nerve

The radial nerve emerges from deep to the tendon of brachioradialis and winds round the radius onto the dorsum of the wrist where it divides into the digital branches of the lateral three and a half digits.

Applied anatomy

As both the ulnar and median nerve give rise to superficial branches which supply the proximal parts of the palm, these branches need to be blocked separately when using wrist blocks.

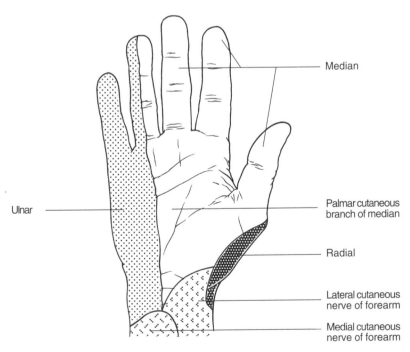

Fig. 2.5.1
Innervation of the hand, palmar view

Ulnar

Median

Palmar cutaneous branch of median

Radial

Lateral cutaneous nerve of forearm

Medial cutaneous nerve of forearm

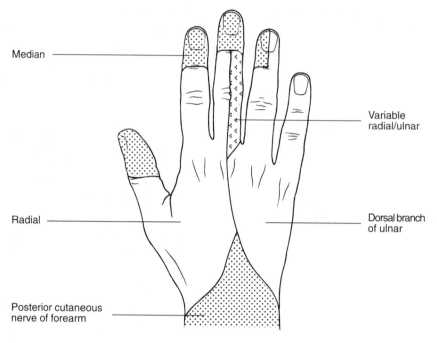

Median

Variable
radial/ulnar

Radial

Dorsal branch
of ulnar

Posterior cutaneous
nerve of forearm

Fig. 2.5.2
Innervation of the hand, dorsal view

Palmar surface of the hand

The skin and deep structures of the palmar
aspect of the hand are innervated by the median
(C6, 7, 8) and ulnar (C8, T1) nerves.

Median nerve

The median nerve divides into its muscular
branch (to the thenar muscles) and common
digital branches as it emerges from the flexor
retinaculum. The sensory nerves in turn divide
at the level of the metacarpo-phalangeal joints
to form the digital nerves to the lateral three and
a half digits (Figs 2.5.1, 2.5.2). The median nerve
gives off a superficial palmar cutaneous branch
just proximal to the flexor retinaculum which
supplies the skin of the thenar eminence and the
palm.

Ulnar nerve

The ulnar nerve accompanies the ulnar artery as
it enters the hand and divides into a deep
branch (which supplies the intrinsic muscles
and other deep structures) and a superficial
branch which gives rise to the common and
then terminal digital nerves to the medial one
and a half digits.

Applied anatomy

If surgery is limited to just one or two adjacent
fingers, then web space blocks (pp. 138–139) are
preferable to a median or ulnar nerve block. For
more extensive surgery, both nerves can be
blocked at the elbow or the wrist depending on
the surgical requirements.

If the proposed surgery involves a skin
incision in the palm of the hand, the median
nerve is better blocked at the elbow as this will
ensure that the palmar cutaneous branch is
blocked. Otherwise the branch needs to be
blocked separately at the wrist as part of the
wrist block.

Dorsal surface of the hand

The dorsum of the hand has a complex and
variable innervation (Fig. 2.5.2) with
contributions from the ulnar, radial and median
nerves.

Ulnar nerve

The ulnar nerve possesses a dorsal branch
which arises about 5 cm proximal to the wrist
on the medial side whence it passes dorsally to
terminate in the dorsal digital nerves of the little

and ring fingers. The dorsal branch sometimes innervates the dorsal aspect of the adjacent side of the middle finger either completely or in conjunction with the radial nerve.

Median nerve

The median nerve innervates a variable area on the dorsal surface of the lateral three and a half digits from the palmar digital nerves.

Radial nerve

The radial nerve terminates on the dorsum of the hand in four or five digital branches which supply the dorsal aspects of the thumb, index finger and the adjacent side of the middle finger. The lateral side of the middle finger is variably supplied by either the ulnar, the radial or both nerves.

Applied anatomy

If the ulnar nerve is blocked at the wrist, the dorsal branch must be blocked separately. This is best done by the medial approach to the ulnar nerve rather than the ventral approach (pp. 126–129). If surgery is limited to the fingers only, then web space blocks are preferable to more proximal blocks (unless more than one finger requires surgery) because of the variable nerve supply. For surgery to multiple fingers the appropriate nerve territories should be blocked at the elbow or wrist as necessary.

Fingers

Digital nerves

The palmar aspect of each digit is supplied by two digital nerves which are derived from either the ulnar (5th finger and ulnar side of ring finger) or the median nerve (radial side of the ring finger, 2nd and 3rd fingers and thumb). These palmar digital nerves also innervate the dorsal aspect of the finger tips and nail beds.

The dorsal digital nerves are similar and derive from either the ulnar nerve (5th and ring finger) or the radial nerve (thumb and 2nd and 3rd fingers). They innervate the skin as far as the distal interphalangeal joint.

There is considerable variation in the exact cutaneous territories supplied by each digital nerve especially at the boundaries of the three parent nerves.

INDICATIONS

- Minor hand surgery – Nerve blocks, either at the wrist or at the digital nerves are suitable for a variety of minor operations including the debridement and suturing of lacerations.
- Complex hand surgery – The nerves to the hand can be blocked either at the elbow or wrist according to the precise requirements of the operation. As with forearm surgery, if a tourniquet is necessary, brachial plexus anaesthesia may be the best option, unless general anaesthesia is to be given. Regional blocks at the wrist provide complete motor and sensory blockade of the hand whilst leaving the flexor and extensor muscles of the forearm unaffected. This can be of advantage in some forms of hand surgery where the patient remains able to move forearm muscles, a situation which aids tendon identification.
- Post-operative analgesia – If a brachial plexus block is to be used for surgical anaesthesia, a short duration local anaesthetic can be used to produce rapid onset and recovery while individual nerves can be blocked distally with a long acting local anaesthetic agent to provide prolonged analgesia in the hand. This allows the patient to regain control of the limb soon after surgery whilst the hand remains pain free for many hours.

Head and neck

Introduction

Regional anaesthesia of the head and neck is infrequently employed by anaesthetists, despite the fact that for both operative anaesthesia and post-operative analgesia, the sensory nerves are easy to locate and block for minor surgery. Increasingly, however, anaesthetists are becoming involved in providing regional anaesthesia for ophthalmic surgery – an area of rapid development in both surgical and anaesthetic techniques. Major surgery to the head and neck for cancer or reconstruction does not lend itself to regional anaesthesia although severe chronic pain states, both malignant and benign, may respond well to diagnostic and neurolytic blocks.

The head and neck are richly innervated by both cranial nerves (CN) and peripheral nerves and the complexity of the nerve supply can be daunting when deciding which specific nerve blocks are appropriate. The majority of cranial nerves have specialised functions and are not considered further in this volume.

Discrete nerve blocks of the pharynx and larynx (CN IX and X) for awake intubation and bronchoscopy have been largely superseded by intraoral topical anaesthesia supplemented by cricothyroid membrane puncture and intratracheal spray.

Cranial nerves

Five of the twelve cranial nerves require practical consideration; the trigeminal nerve (CN V) has somatic cutaneous nerve fibres which innervate the anterior two-thirds of the scalp and the face (Fig. 2.6.1). It also has motor function and controls the muscles of mastication. The facial nerve (CN VII) is entirely motor (apart from its secretory and taste function) and controls the muscles of facial expression. The three cranial nerves which control the extraocular muscles are the oculomotor, the trochlear and the abducens (CN III, IV and VI) and can be considered as a single entity for ophthalmic surgery.

Trigeminal nerve

The trigeminal nerve has three divisions; ophthalmic (V1), maxillary (V2) and mandibular (V3) which terminate in eleven cutaneous nerves (Figs 2.6.1, 2.6.2). Of these, the supraorbital and supratrochlear (V1), the infraorbital, zygomaticofacial and zygomaticotemporal (V2) and the mental (V3) all emerge from foramina or bony notches which can be palpated and the nerves blocked by discrete injection (pp. 146–149).

The external nasal, infratrochlear (branches of the nasociliary) and lacrimal nerves (all V1) arise within the margins of the orbit.

The supraorbital and supratrochlear nerves can be considered together as they are both terminal nerves of V1 and they emerge close together at the superior and superiomedial borders of the orbit to supply the skin of the upper eyelid and lower forehead (supratrochlear) and the forehead and the anterior aspect of the scalp as far back as the vertex (supraorbital).

The infraorbital nerve emerges from the infraorbital foramen about 1 cm below the midpoint of the lower orbital border. It innervates the skin of the lower eyelid, side of the nose, cheek and upper lip (Fig. 2.6.3).

The zygomaticofacial and zygomatico-temporal nerves emerge from small foraminae in the anterior and temporal parts of the zygoma, near the orbital margin, to supply the skin of the cheek prominence, temple and temporal scalp (Fig. 2.6.3).

The mental nerve emerges from the mental foramen in the mandible to innervate the skin of the chin and lower lip (Fig. 2.6.3).

The auriculotemporal nerve emerges from behind the temporomandibular joint and accompanies the superficial temporal artery which serves as a convenient landmark. Its superficial temporal branches innervate the skin of the temple and an anterior auricular branch innervates the skin of the tragus and part of the helix of the ear (Fig. 2.6.3).

Applied anatomy

The supraorbital, infraorbital and mental foraminae lie in the same vertical plane which runs through the pupil when the eye is in the primary mid position.

Ophthalmic

Maxillary

Mandibular

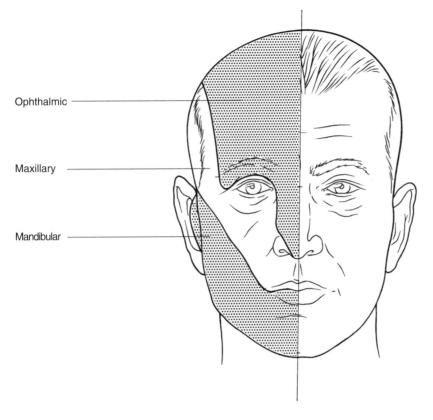

Fig. 2.6.1
Divisions of the trigeminal nerve

Supraorbital
Supratrochlear

Zygomaticofacial
Zygomaticotemporal

Infraorbital

Mental

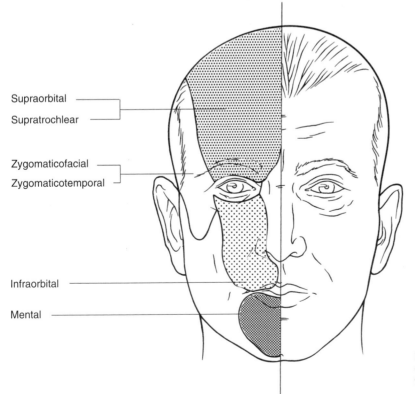

Fig. 2.6.2
Cranial nerves innervating the face

Facial nerve

The facial nerve divides within the parotid gland into its five terminal branches which are all motor to the intrinsic muscles of the face. In particular, the temporal and zygomatic branches which supply the orbicularis oculi muscles are of importance for ophthalmic procedures. The nerves emerge from the parotid gland immediately anterior to the tragus and cross the zygomatic arch towards the temple and lateral border of the orbit.

Cervical nerves

The first four cervical nerves innervate the posterior aspect of the scalp as far forward as the vertex, the inferior and posterior surfaces of the ear and the neck. The dorsal rami of C1 and C2 are large in comparison to the ventral rami and form the suboccipital (C1), which is motor only, and greater occipital (C2) nerves which supply the scalp. The dorsal rami of C3 and C4 innervate the skin of the back of the neck (Fig. 2.6.4).

Greater occipital nerve

The greater occipital nerve ascends the posterior aspect of the neck and pierces the trapezius muscle about 2 cm lateral to the occipital protuberance to become subcutaneous. It is accompanied by the occipital artery, which acts as a landmark for identification. It innervates the scalp as far anterior as the vertex and often communicates with the lesser occipital nerve.

Applied anatomy

The greater and lesser occipital nerves supply the adjacent parts of the scalp and often communicate with each other, therefore they need to be blocked together to provide complete analgesia of the posterior aspect of the scalp.

The ventral rami of C1–4 combine to form the cervical plexus anterior to the scalenus medius muscle and deep to the sternomastoid muscle and internal jugular vein. The plexus gives rise to both superficial and deep branches which can be separated functionally and anatomically. The deep branches of the plexus are all motor with the exception of the phrenic nerve which has efferent visceral sensory nerve fibres.

Superficial cervical plexus

The superficial branches of the plexus (C2–4) are cutaneous and emerge from behind the posterior border of sternomastoid muscle at its midpoint (Fig. 2.6.5). They penetrate the superficial leaf of the deep cervical fascia and then radiate out subcutaneously to supply the ear and surrounding skin of the scalp and face (lesser occipital and greater auricular nerves), the skin of the submandibular area, the neck and 'cape' area, i.e. the anterior and posterior aspects of the shoulder, and the uppermost parts of the chest wall (the anterior cutaneous nerve and the supraclavicular nerves).

Deep cervical plexus

The cervical roots emerge from the intervertebral foraminae and lie in the sulcus of the transverse processes before they combine to form the plexus. Thus, any approach to the roots is, in effect, a cervical paravertebral block.

Applied anatomy

There are few indications for a deep approach to the cervical plexus as all the deep branches are motor. In addition, any injection made at the level of the roots will produce phrenic nerve paralysis and may spread to the more distal cervical nerves causing a partial brachial plexus block. Limiting cervical plexus blocks to the superficial branches achieves complete sensory blockade without motor deficit and the potentially serious complications of vertebral artery or epidural injection are avoided.

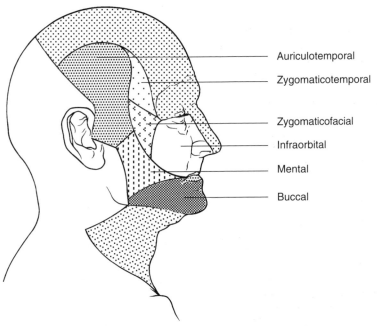

Fig. 2.6.3
Cranially sourced nerves innervating the head and neck

Auriculotemporal

Zygomaticotemporal

Zygomaticofacial

Infraorbital

Mental

Buccal

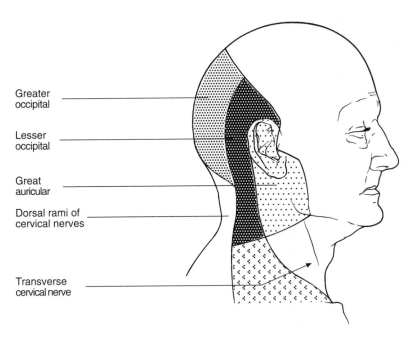

Greater occipital

Lesser occipital

Great auricular

Dorsal rami of cervical nerves

Transverse cervical nerve

Fig. 2.6.4
Peripheral nerves innervating the head and neck

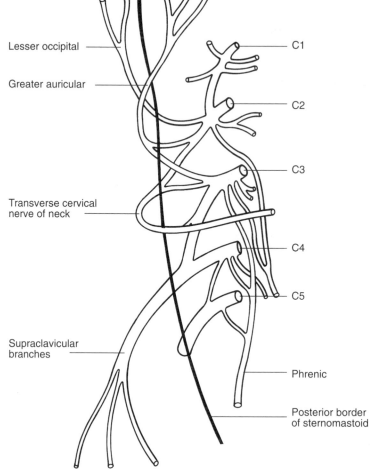

Fig. 2.6.5
Superficial cervical plexus

Labels on figure:
- Lesser occipital
- Greater auricular
- Transverse cervical nerve of neck
- Supraclavicular branches
- C1
- C2
- C3
- C4
- C5
- Phrenic
- Posterior border of sternomastoid

Suprascapular nerve

Although the suprascapular nerve is a branch of the brachial plexus it can be considered as a derivative of the cervical nerves (C5, 6) and may be blocked in conjunction with the cervical plexus for operations on the shoulder. It arises from the upper trunk of the brachial plexus and passes through the suprascapular notch of the scapula to lie deep to the supraspinatus muscle where it innervates the shoulder joint (rotator cuff and glenoid) and the acromioclavicular joint.

Many operations on the head and neck can be carried out under local anaesthesia alone or regional techniques can be employed to supplement general anaesthesia.

INDICATIONS

- Surgery of the scalp – Wounds of the scalp can be repaired under a combination of nerve blocks according to the position of the wound. Posterior to the ears, the greater and lesser occipital and great auricular nerves need to be blocked. Anterior to the ears, the supratrochlear, supraorbital and auriculotemporal nerves need to be blocked as appropriate.
- Surgery of the face – Superficial surgery to the face can be accomplished with discrete nerve blocks of the appropriate nerve(s), supplemented as necessary with local infiltration.
- Surgery of the ear – Plastic or other external operations on the ears can be

carried out with blockade of the auriculotemporal nerve anteriorly and the greater auricular and lesser occipital nerves posteriorly.

- Surgery of the neck – Most surgery only requires superficial cervical plexus blockade. Bilateral blocks are required for midline operations such as tracheostomy and thyroidectomy and may need to be reinforced with deeper local infiltration. Deep cervical plexus block has been advocated for these procedures but in view of the need for bilateral blocks and the risk of bilateral phrenic nerve blockade, this cannot be recommended. Deep cervical plexus blocks have been used successfully for carotid arterial surgery (for example endarterectomy) but this remains a controversial technique.

Head and neck

Indications

Ophthalmology

Introduction

The majority of operations within the orbit can be accomplished under regional anaesthesia. In particular, cataract surgery is now routinely carried out under regional anaesthesia in day stay surgical units in many centres. Regional anaesthesia for ophthalmic surgery may be administered by either surgeon or anaesthetist provided that they receive appropriate training in performing the techniques and are fully conversant with the associated risks and complications and can treat them accordingly.

Orbit

The orbit contains the eyeball (globe), the six extraocular muscles, the lacrimal gland and the associated nerve and blood supplies. The surrounding structures of the orbital margins are supplied by vessels and nerves that traverse the orbit. The only structure involved in operations on the eye which requires separate anaesthesia outside the orbital margins is the orbicularis oculi muscle of the eyelids.

Extraocular muscles

There are seven extraocular muscles in total; one controls the upper eyelid (levator palpebrae superioris) and six control movement of the globe. The four rectus muscles (superior, inferior, medial and lateral) arise from a common tendon around the optic foramen and form a cone of muscle as they pass forward to their insertions on the globe. Within the cone are: the ophthalmic artery, the ciliary ganglion and the optic (CN II), oculomotor (CN III), abducens (CN VI) and nasociliary (CN V) nerves whilst the trochlear (CN IV), lacrimal, frontal and infraorbital (all CN V) remain outside the cone.

The orbit and its contents receive a complex innervation of motor, sensory and autonomic nerves (Table 2.3).

Applied anatomy

The cone of extraocular muscles forms a boundary which defines the differences between the techniques and effects of the

Table 2.3 Innervation of the orbit and its contents

Modality	Nerve	Innervation
motor	oculomotor (CN III)	superior rectus medial rectus inferior oblique
	trochlear (CN IV)	superior oblique
	abducens (CN VI)	lateral rectus
	facial (CN VII)	orbicularis oculi
sensory	trigeminal (CN V)	
	ophthalmic division	
	supratrochlear	skin/conjunctiva upper lid
	supraorbital	skin/conjunctiva upper lid
	long ciliary	cornea, iris, ciliary muscle
	nasociliary/infratrochlear	inner eyelids, inner canthus
	lacrimal	lateral canthus, gland, outer lid, conjunctiva
	maxillary division	
	infraorbital	lower lid, nasolacrimal duct
	zygomatic	lateral wall of orbit
autonomic	sympathetic long and short ciliary nerves from superior cervical ganglion	iris dilation
	para-sympathetic fibres from CN III	iris constriction

peribulbar and retrobulbar blocks. With the former, the local anaesthetic solution is injected outside the cone; with the latter, it is injected within the cone. Due to the small volume of the cone, a retrobulbar injection will generate a higher pressure than an equivalent volume injected into the peribulbar space. Similarly, a retrobulbar injection works more quickly than a peribulbar injection because the local anaesthetic is placed directly onto the nerves within the cone. When using a retrobulbar block, the intention is to place the needle tip behind the globe so it is necessary to know the axial diameter of the globe. The average diameter is 24 mm but in myopic patients the diameter may be greater than this and, because the sclera is thinner in these elongated eyes, retrobulbar blocks are contraindicated if the eye diameter is greater than 25 mm.

conjunctival instillation of local anaesthetic solution provides effective post-operative analgesia.

INDICATIONS

- Corneal/conjunctival surgery – Minor surgery to the cornea, sclera and conjunctiva can be carried out under topical anaesthesia alone or in combination with a subconjunctival injection. Such surgery might include: intraocular pressure measurement, removal of foreign bodies, excision of pterygium, irrigation of the lacrimal duct and removal of sutures. Surgical correction of myopia (radial keratotomy) may be undertaken using topical anaesthesia. The increasing use of phakoemulsification for the removal of cataract through a small limbic incision and the development of very flexible intraocular lenses, makes it possible to perform major intraocular surgery under topical anaesthesia alone.
- Intraocular surgery – This requires sensory blockade of the globe and conjunctiva with motor blockade of the extraocular and periorbital muscles so that the operative site is immobile, the pupil is dilated and the intraocular pressure low. Extracapsular extraction of cataract and insertion of an intraocular lens is the most common procedure carried out under regional anaesthesia but other procedures are equally feasible.
- Extraocular surgery – The correction of squint is normally performed under general anaesthesia but pre-operative

Techniques

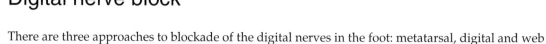

Digital nerve block

There are three approaches to blockade of the digital nerves in the foot: metatarsal, digital and web space.

Metatarsal block

Landmarks
   Intermetatarsal spaces

Metatarsal block is useful when anaesthesia of the intrinsic muscles and other deep structures of the forefoot is required in addition to cutaneous analgesia of the toes. Identify the spaces between the metatarsals which correspond to the toes to be blocked at the midpoint of the metatarsal bones (halfway down the dorsum of the foot). Insert a 22 G short bevel needle vertically downwards aiming towards the plantar surface of the foot. Place a palpating finger on the sole which will detect the needle approaching the deep plantar fascia,

as shown in Figure 3.1.1. The needle should *not* penetrate the plantar fascia as the digital nerves lie above it. Inject 2 ml of solution, withdraw the needle slowly while injecting a further 2 ml and finally inject 2 ml at the level of the dorsal surface of the metatarsal bone (Figs 3.1.1, 3.1.2).

Agent	Concn	Volume	Onset	Duration
Bupiv	0.5%	6 ml	20 min	6–12 h
Lido	1%	6 ml	5 min	3 h

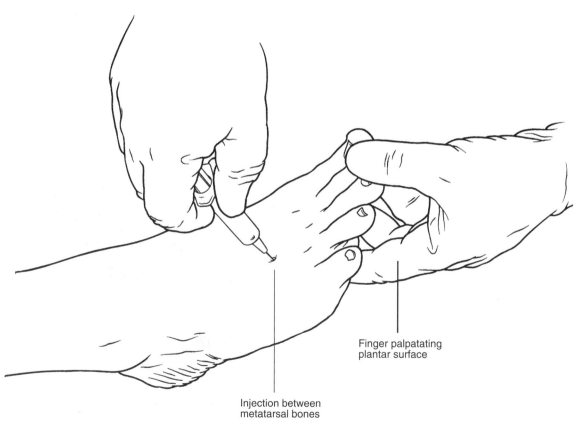

Finger palpatating
plantar surface

Injection between
metatarsal bones

Fig. 3.1.1
Metatarsal block

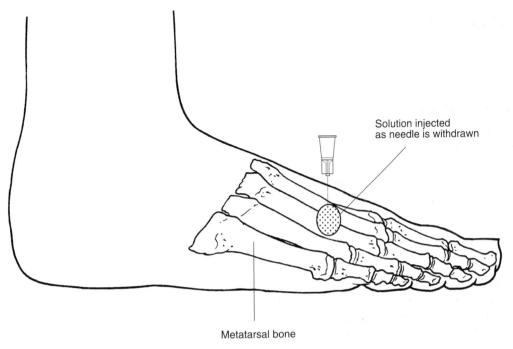

Solution injected
as needle is withdrawn

Metatarsal bone

Fig. 3.1.2
Metatarsal block, lateral view

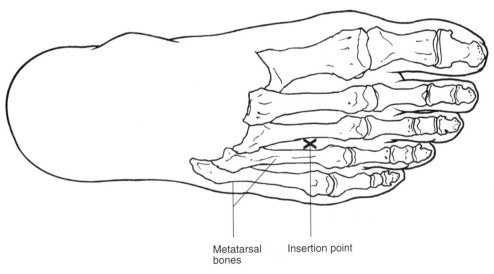

Metatarsal
bones

Insertion point

Fig. 3.1.3
Metatarsal block, superior view

Technique   **57**

Digital nerve block

Landmarks
  Metatarso-phalangeal joints
  Web spaces

When analgesia of the toes alone is desired, the digital nerves can be blocked at the level of the metatarso-phalangeal joints either side of the appropriate toe(s). Insert a 22 G short bevel needle vertically downwards at a point above the web space, just distal to the metatarso-phalangeal joint. Place a finger under the plantar surface of the web space to detect the approaching needle tip as it reaches the plantar border of the proximal phalanx (Fig. 3.2.1). Stop and withdraw the needle slowly whilst injecting 3 ml of solution (Figs 3.2.2, 3.2.3).

Agent	Concn	Volume	Onset	Duration
Bupiv	0.5%	3 ml	20 min	6–12 h
Lido	1%	3 ml	5 min	3 h

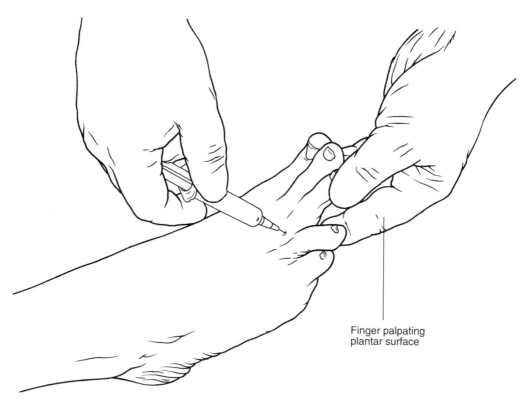

Finger palpating
plantar surface

Fig. 3.2.1
Digital nerve block

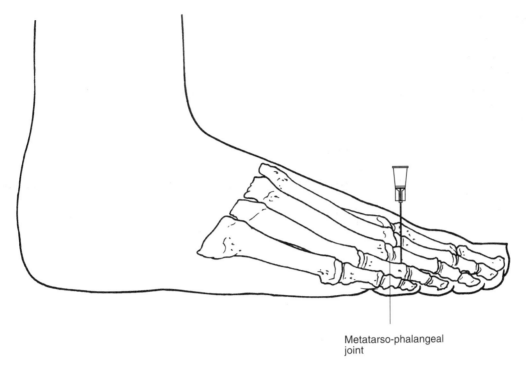

Metatarso-phalangeal
joint

Fig. 3.2.2
Digital nerve block, lateral view

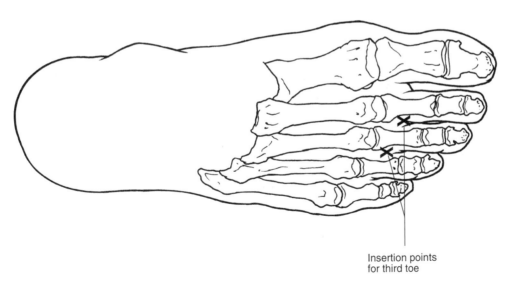

Insertion points
for third toe

Fig. 3.2.3
Digital nerve block, superior view

Web space block

Landmarks
  Web spaces

An approach in the horizontal plane (cf. previous technique). Separate the toes that delimit the web space as in Figure 3.3.1 and insert a 23 G needle into the web space to a depth of 2 cm until the needle tip is level with the metatarso-phalangeal joint (Figs 3.3.2, 3.3.3). Inject 4 ml of solution. There should be no resistance to injection and the web space will distend slightly. Gentle massage of the distended space will disperse the solution around both dorsal and plantar digital nerves. In the conscious patient, web space block is the least uncomfortable technique (especially if a 25 G or 27 G needle is used).

Note. To avoid precipitating ischaemia, solutions containing vasoconstrictors *should not be used*. High pressure within the confines of a web space, produced by excessive volume of injectate, must also be avoided. Limit volume to 4 ml of solution per web space.

Agent	Concn	Volume	Onset	Duration
Bupiv	0.5%	4 ml	30 min	6–12 h
Lido	1%	4 ml	5 min	3 h

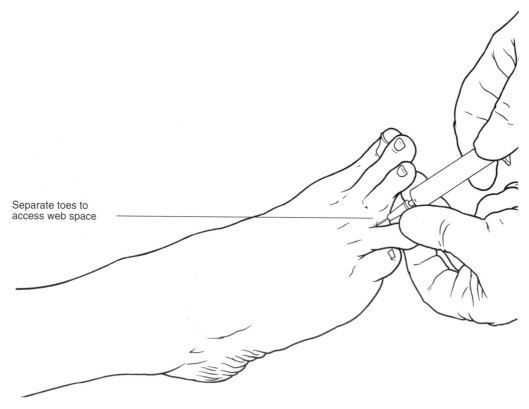

Separate toes to access web space

Fig. 3.3.1
Web space block

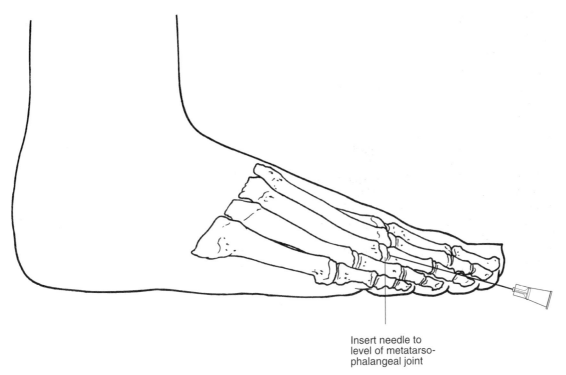

Insert needle to
level of metatarso-
phalangeal joint

Fig. 3.3.2
Web space block, lateral view

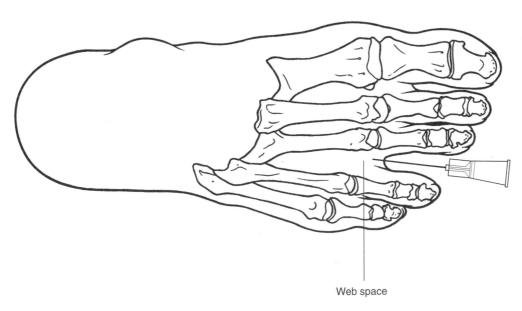

Web space

Fig. 3.3.3
Web space block, superior view

Sural nerve block

Landmarks
    Achilles tendon
    Lateral malleolus

Position the patient supine with the foot inverted. Insert a 22 G short bevel needle behind the lateral malleolus aiming for the lateral border of the Achilles tendon as in Figure 3.4.1. If paraesthesiae occur, inject 5 ml of solution. Paraesthesiae may not be elicited because the nerve has usually divided into several branches at this level. It is thus more effective if a subcutaneous 'sausage' of solution is injected between the malleolus and the Achilles tendon to block all branches (Fig. 3.4.2).

Agent	Concn	Volume	Onset	Duration
Bupiv	0.5%	5 ml	20 min	6–12 h
Prilo	1%	5 ml	10 min	4 h
Lido	1%	5 ml	5 min	3 h

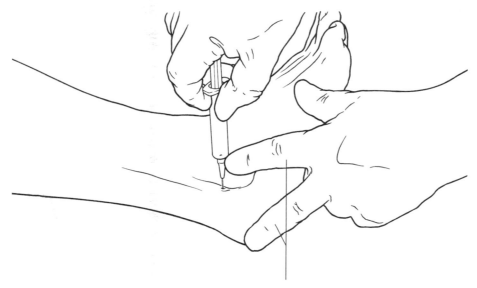

Fingers indicating landmarks

Fig. 3.4.1
Sural nerve block

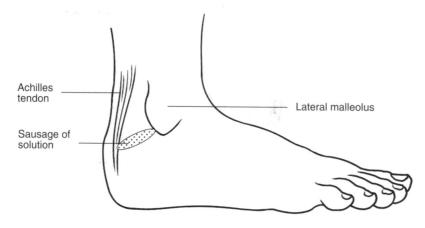

Achilles tendon

Sausage of solution

Lateral malleolus

Fig. 3.4.2
Sural nerve block, lateral view

Saphenous nerve block

Landmarks
Medial malleolus
Long saphenous vein

Externally rotate the leg with the patient lying supine. Identify the long saphenous vein. Venous occlusion can be used to bring it into prominence. At a point 1 cm proximal and 1 cm anterior to the medial malleolus, inject 5 ml of solution in a subcutaneous infiltration around the vein. Avoid intravenous injection (Fig. 3.5.1).

Agent	Concn	Volume	Onset	Duration
Bupiv	0.5%	3–5 ml	20 min	6–12 h
Prilo	1%	3–5 ml	10 min	4 h
Lido	1%	3–5 ml	5 min	3 h

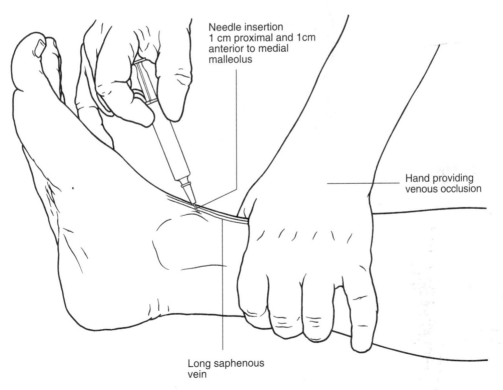

Needle insertion 1 cm proximal and 1cm anterior to medial malleolus

Hand providing venous occlusion

Long saphenous vein

Fig. 3.5.1
Saphenous nerve block

Peroneal nerve block

Deep peroneal nerve

Landmarks
   Extensor digitorum longus tendons
   Extensor hallucis longus tendon
   Dorsalis pedis pulsation

The natural skin crease across the dorsum of the foot corresponds to a line joining the malleoli. At this level the dorsalis pedis pulse can be palpated between the extensor hallucis longus tendon medially, and the extensor digitorum longus tendons laterally. With the foot supported in extension, insert a 23 G needle just medial to the pulsation of the dorsalis pedis as in Figure 3.6.1. Advance the needle 1 cm forward. If bone is struck or resistance to further movement is felt (indicating that the needle may be in a tendon or tendon sheath) withdraw and reposition (Fig. 3.6.3).

Agent	Concn	Volume	Onset	Duration
Bupiv	0.5%	5 ml	20 min	6–12 h
Prilo	1%	5 ml	10 min	4 h
Lido	1%	5 ml	5 min	3 h

Superficial peroneal nerve

Landmarks
  As for deep peroneal nerve

It is usual to block the superficial and deep peroneal nerves in combination. After completion of the deep block, withdraw the needle to the subcutaneous plane and re-angle laterally. Inject a 7 ml 'sausage' of solution as the needle is advanced laterally along a line parallel to the line joining the two malleoli (Figs 3.6.2, 3.6.4).

Agent	Concn	Volume	Onset	Duration
Bupiv	0.5%	5 ml	20 min	6–12 h
Prilo	1%	5 ml	10 min	4 h
Lido	1%	5 ml	5 min	3 h

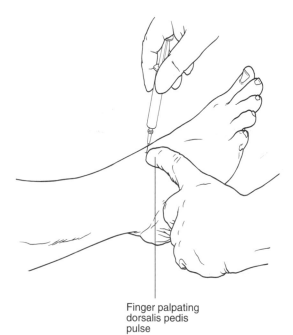

Finger palpating
dorsalis pedis
pulse

Fig. 3.6.1
Deep peroneal nerve block

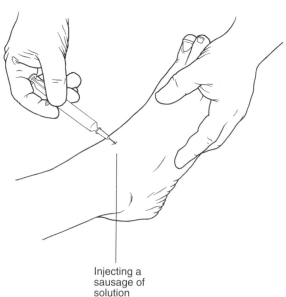

Injecting a
sausage of
solution

Fig. 3.6.2
Superficial peroneal nerve block

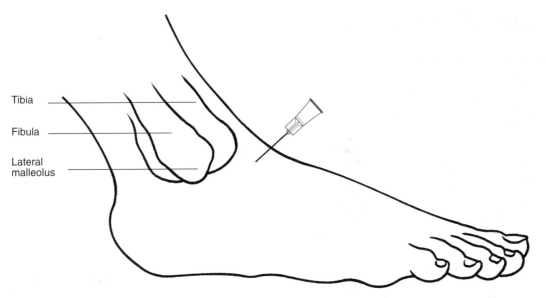

Fig. 3.6.3
Deep peroneal block, lateral view

Tibia

Fibula

Lateral malleolus

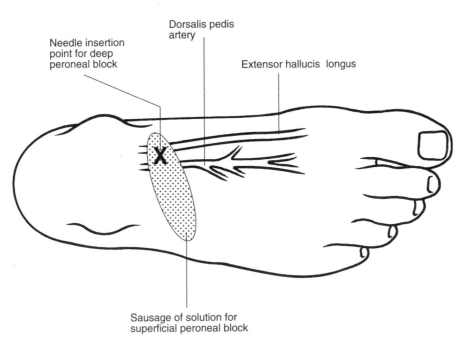

Needle insertion point for deep peroneal block

Dorsalis pedis artery

Extensor hallucis longus

X

Sausage of solution for superficial peroneal block

Fig. 3.6.4
Peroneal nerve block, superior view

Tibial nerve block

There are two approaches to the tibial nerve at the level of the medial malleolus, classical and sustentaculum tali.

Classical approach

Landmarks
   Medial malleolus
   Tibial artery pulsation
   Periosteum of calcaneum

Place the leg in the 'figure of four' position. Palpate the pulsation of the posterior tibial artery and leave the finger in position. From a point immediately behind the medial malleolus, insert a 22 G short bevel needle parallel to the tibia as in Figure 3.7.1, towards the palpating finger and deep to the pulsation. The conscious patient will usually feel paraesthesiae just prior to the needle striking the periosteum of the calcaneum. Ensure that the needle tip is not subperiosteal by withdrawing 2 mm (Figs 3.7.2, 3.7.3).

Agent	Concn	Volume	Onset	Duration
Bupiv	0.5%	6 ml	20 min	6–12 h
Prilo	1%	6 ml	10 min	4 h
Lido	1%	6 ml	5 min	3 h

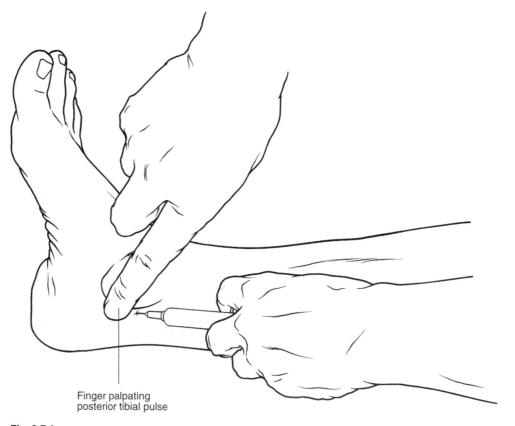

Finger palpating
posterior tibial pulse

Fig. 3.7.1
Tibial nerve block (classical approach)

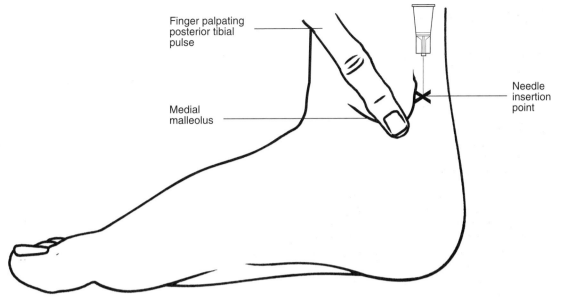

Finger palpating
posterior tibial
pulse

Medial
malleolus

Needle
insertion
point

Fig. 3.7.2
Tibial nerve block, medial view

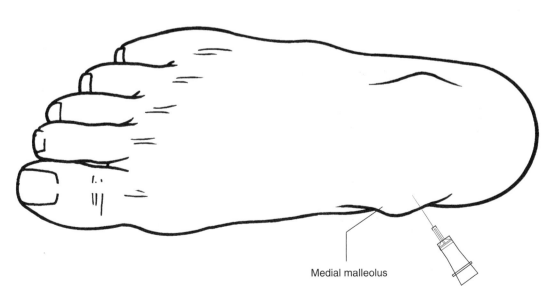

Medial malleolus

Fig. 3.7.3
Tibial nerve block, superior view

Technique   **67**

Sustentaculum tali approach

Landmarks
 Sustentaculum tali
 Medial border of heel
 Flexor retinaculum

Position patient in 'figure of four'. Identify the distal end of the medial malleolus. A ridge of bone, the sustentaculum tali, may be felt 1 cm distal to the malleolus. At a point midway between this ridge and the medial border of the heel, insert a 22 G short bevel needle as in Figure 3.8.1. Penetration of the flexor retinaculum will be felt as a 'pop'. Paraesthesiae may be felt by the patient but the injection may be made without this sign. Injection should be easy with little resistance to flow.

A subcutaneous swelling indicates that the retinaculum has not been penetrated and the needle should be re-positioned more deeply (Figs 3.8.2, 3.8.3).

Agent	Concn	Volume	Onset	Duration
Bupiv	0.5%	8 ml	20 min	6–12 h
Prilo	1%	8 ml	10 min	4 h
Lido	1%	8 ml	5 min	3 h

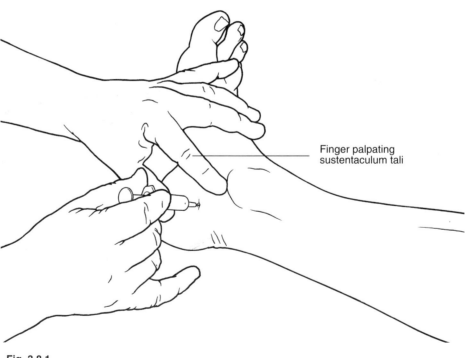

Finger palpating sustentaculum tali

Fig. 3.8.1
Tibial nerve block (sustentaculum tali approach)

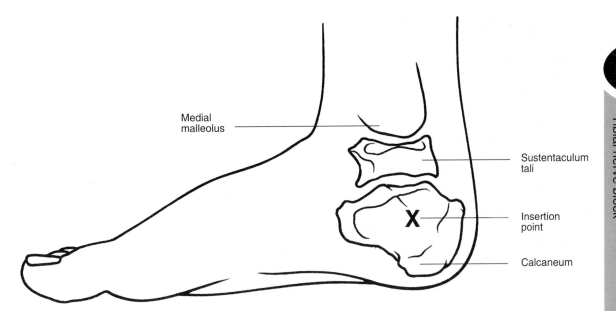

Fig. 3.8.2
Tibial nerve block, medial view

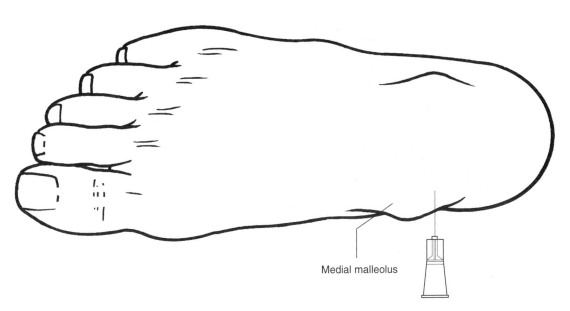

Fig. 3.8.3
Tibial nerve block, superior view

Saphenous nerve block

There are two approaches to the saphenous nerve. The proximal approach is described below and the distal approach is described in the foot section (p. 63).

Proximal approach

Landmarks
Medial condyle of tibia
Tibial tuberosity

Externally rotate the leg with the patient in the supine position and identify the bony prominence of the medial tibial condyle. The saphenous nerve is accessible at this level and can therefore be blocked by injecting a 'sausage' of solution from the anterior aspect of the condyle towards its posterior border. Insert a 23 G needle 2 cm postero-medial to the tibial tuberosity, as in Figure 3.9.1, keeping in the subcutaneous plane. Inject as the needle is advanced towards the posterior of the condyle (Figs 3.9.2, 3.9.3).

Agent	Concn	Volume	Onset	Duration
Bupiv	0.5%	10–15 ml	15 min	6–8 h

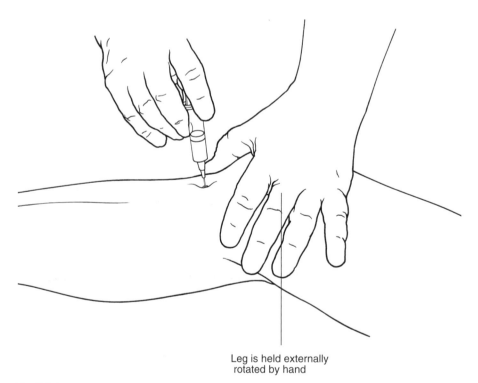

Leg is held externally
rotated by hand

Fig. 3.9.1
Saphenous nerve block

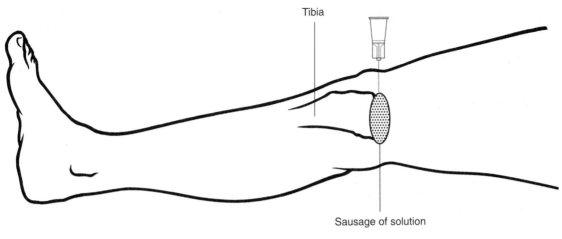

Tibia

Sausage of solution

Fig. 3.9.2
Saphenous nerve block, medial view

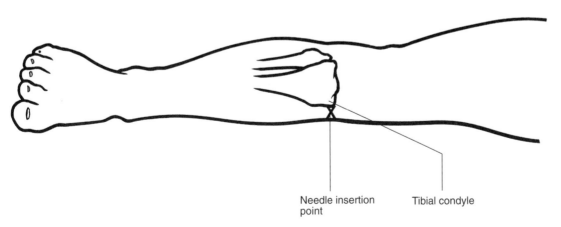

Needle insertion
point

Tibial condyle

Fig. 3.9.3
Saphenous nerve block, anterior view

Popliteal fossa block

The sciatic nerve and its two principal terminal branches (peroneal and tibial nerves) can be blocked by a single injection into the popliteal fossa. For complete anaesthesia below the knee, a combined technique with a saphenous nerve block at the knee (pp. 70–71) is necessary. Popliteal fossa block is easy to perform, especially with a peripheral nerve stimulator, but requires a prone patient and is therefore best suited to the conscious patient.

Landmarks
   Posterior skin crease of knee joint
   Popliteal artery pulse

Position the patient prone and define the popliteal fossa by identifying the tendinous insertions of the hamstring muscles above and the origins of the gastrocnemius muscle heads below. The posterior skin crease of the knee joint marks the widest point of the popliteal fossa and at this point with the knee slightly flexed, the popliteal pulse can be palpated. Just lateral to the pulsation and 2–3 cm above the skin crease, insert a 22 G short bevel needle (Fig. 3.10.1). Advance 2–3 cm, taking care to avoid intravascular placement. Paraesthesiae in the lower leg indicate correct positioning. Alternatively, a peripheral nerve stimulator can be employed to evoke peroneal nerve activity which will produce dorsiflexion and eversion of the foot (if the tibial nerve is stimulated, plantar flexion and inversion will be seen). For a large knee, a longer needle will be necessary as the nerves may lie up to 4 cm deep. It may also be necessary to insert the needle in a superior, oblique direction to seek the nerves higher up in the fossa. After aspiration, inject 10–15 ml of solution. There should be little resistance to the flow of solution (Figs 3.10.2, 3.10.3).

Agent	Concn	Volume	Onset	Duration
Bupiv	0.5%	10–15 ml	15 min	6–12 h

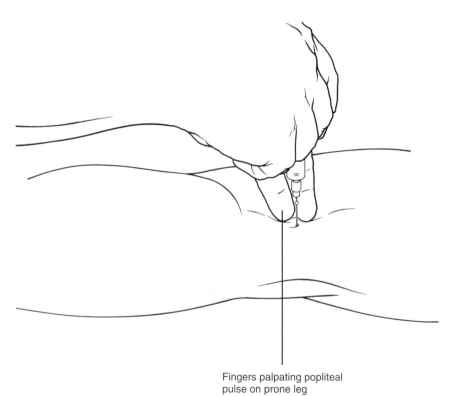

Fingers palpating popliteal
pulse on prone leg

Fig. 3.10.1
Popliteal fossa block

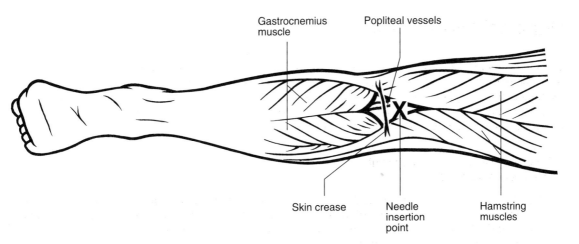

Gastrocnemius muscle

Popliteal vessels

Skin crease

Needle insertion point

Hamstring muscles

Fig. 3.10.2
Popliteal fossa block, posterior view

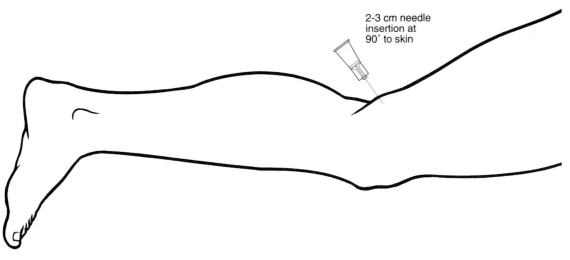

2-3 cm needle insertion at 90° to skin

Fig. 3.10.3
Popliteal fossa block, medial view

Intra-articular block

The increasing use of arthroscopic knee surgery has led to the development of intra-articular anaesthesia which has been shown to be effective both for surgery and post-operative analgesia. There is evidence that the intra-articular injection of morphine improves the quality of analgesia following surgery; this highlights the role of peripheral opioid receptors in inflamed synovial tissue.

Landmarks
  Medial border of patella

Fully extend the leg and identify the gap between the medial border of the patella and the femur. Insert a 22 G short bevel needle into the knee joint, as in Figure 3.11.1, taking care to avoid damaging the articular surfaces. Inject 30 ml of 0.5% bupivacaine with 1: 200 000 adrenaline into the joint, paying regard to the recommended maximum dose (Figs 3.11.2, 3.11.3). After gentle manipulation of the knee, leave the patient resting for a minimum of 20 min. The addition of 1–2 mg of morphine to the local anaesthetic solution has been shown to prolong post-operative analgesia. Immediately prior to surgery, the portals of entry for the surgical instruments should be infiltrated using 1% prilocaine. This is usually undertaken by the surgeon who has the clearest idea of where to insert the instruments. The benefits of this technique are most apparent in day surgery because there is neither cutaneous sensory deficit nor motor weakness and thus the patient can ambulate immediately after the operation. Provided that sufficient time is allowed for the local anaesthetic solution to penetrate the synovium and for the adrenaline to produce full vasoconstriction, relatively major surgery, including meniscectomy, chondroplasty and synovial resection is possible.

Agent	Concn	Volume	Onset	Duration
Bupiv + adren	0.5%	30 ml	45 min	3–5 h

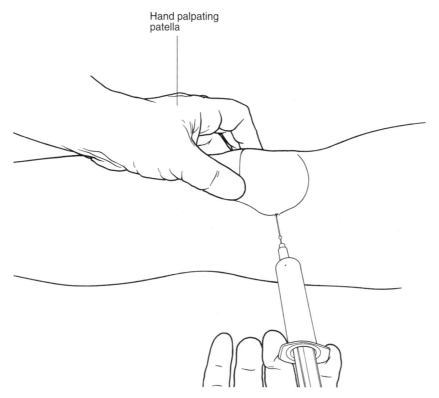

Hand palpating patella

Fig. 3.11.1
Intra-articular block of the knee

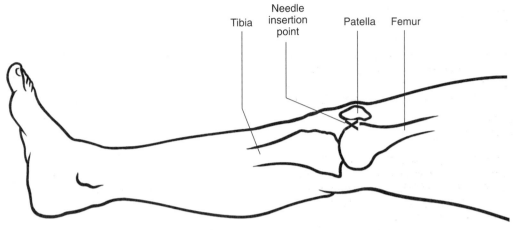

Fig. 3.11.2
Intra-articular block of the knee, medial view

Tibia Needle insertion point Patella Femur

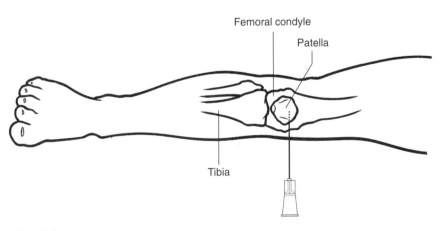

Femoral condyle Patella Tibia

Fig 3.11.3
Intra-articular block of the knee, anterior view

Femoral nerve block

The femoral nerve can be blocked as an individual nerve, using a small volume of solution (10–15 ml). Alternatively, it can be incorporated into a distal approach to the lumbar plexus. This is the so called '3 in 1' block described by Winnie et al (1973) using volumes of 20–30 ml to produce a collective block of the femoral, obturator and lateral cutaneous nerve of thigh.

Controversy. The three nerves are not always reliably blocked by the distal approach via the femoral nerve sheath. The lateral cutaneous nerve of thigh is most frequently missed due to its more proximal position and different nerve root origins within the lumbar plexus. Conversely, because the lumbar plexus contains a major contribution to the sacral plexus – the lumbosacral trunk – a '3 in 1' block may spill over into the sciatic nerve distribution. Thus, this block may range from a '1 in 1' to a '4 in 1' block depending on the volume of local anaesthetic solution injected and anatomical variation within the psoas compartment.

Landmarks
  Inguinal ligament
  Femoral artery

Define the inguinal ligament by drawing a line between the anterior superior iliac spine and the pubic tubercle. Palpate the femoral arterial pulse and, at a point approximately 1 cm lateral to the pulse and 1–2 cm below the inguinal ligament, insert a 22 G short bevel needle as in Figure 3.12.1. Slowly advance. If the bevel of the needle is placed flat on the skin, a greater degree of 'feel' will help to identify two distinct 'pops' as the tip of the needle penetrates firstly the fascia lata and then the ilio-pectineal fascia that invests the nerve. Depending on the amount of superficial fat, the nerve is between 1 and 3 cm deep to the skin. The use of a peripheral nerve stimulator at this stage will assist accurate needle placement because the nerve may not bear such a constant relationship to the artery as is commonly supposed and it can be difficult to locate 'blind' (Figs 3.12.2, 3.12.3). Pulse synchronous movement of the sartorious muscle indicates that the anterior division of the nerve has been located. It is preferable to identify branches of the posterior division, which produce pulse synchronous movement of the patellar mechanism, if motor blockade of the quadriceps muscles and anaesthesia of the knee joint is required. If paraesthesiae are to be used as the end point of nerve location, then they should be sought in the knee joint itself or in the distribution of the saphenous nerve (p. 29) because it is a branch of the posterior division of the femoral nerve.

Note. In view of the close proximity of the femoral vessels, careful aspiration of the syringe is essential prior to injection.

Agent	Concn	Volume	Onset	Duration
Femoral				
Bupiv	0.5%	10–15 ml	30 min	8–12 h
Bupiv	0.75%	10 ml	20 min	12–24 h
'3 in 1' block				
Bupiv	0.5%	30 ml	30 min	8–12 h

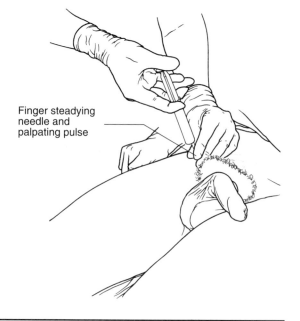

Finger steadying needle and palpating pulse

Fig. 3.12.1
Femoral nerve block

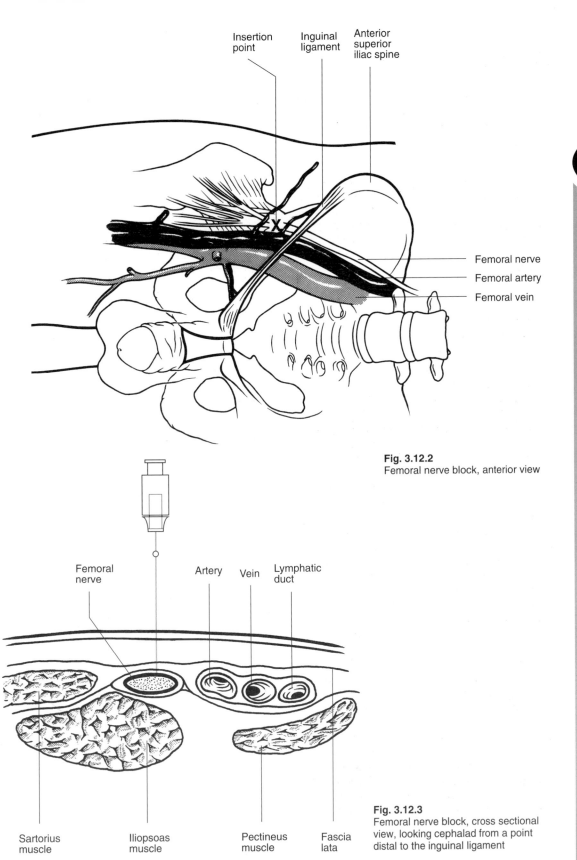

Insertion point

Inguinal ligament

Anterior superior iliac spine

Femoral nerve

Femoral artery

Femoral vein

Fig. 3.12.2
Femoral nerve block, anterior view

Femoral nerve

Artery

Vein

Lymphatic duct

Sartorius muscle

Iliopsoas muscle

Pectineus muscle

Fascia lata

Fig. 3.12.3
Femoral nerve block, cross sectional view, looking cephalad from a point distal to the inguinal ligament

Sciatic nerve block

The sciatic nerve is the largest peripheral nerve in the body and the most deeply situated. In the conscious patient, without the use of a peripheral nerve stimulator, sciatic nerve blocks can be uncomfortable and difficult to perform successfully. In both conscious and anaesthetised patients, the use of a nerve stimulator will improve the accuracy of nerve location and ensure a higher success rate. As the nerve is large, it is important to use a high concentration of local anaesthetic (0.75% bupivacaine or 2% lidocaine) and to be patient about waiting for the block to develop. It may take 45–60 min for full motor and sensory block to occur. There are four proximal approaches to the sciatic nerve. Three only are described here as the lateral approach is technically more difficult and offers no particular advantages. Patient positioning for the classical, lithotomy and anterior approaches are shown in Figures 3.13.1, 3.13.2 and 3.13.3 respectively.

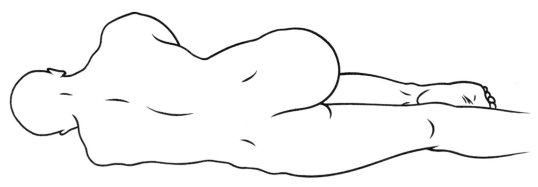

Fig. 3.13.1
Sciatic nerve block, classical approach

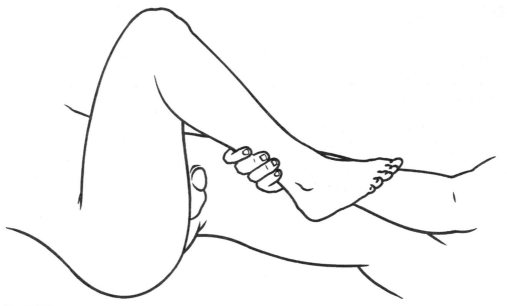

Fig. 3.13.2
Sciatic nerve block, lithotomy approach

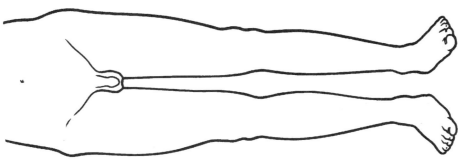

Fig. 3.13.3
Sciatic nerve block, anterior approach

Classical approach of Labat

Landmarks
- Posterior superior iliac spine
- Sacro-coccygeal joint
- Greater trochanter

Position the patient in the lateral position, with the side to be blocked uppermost. Extend the bottom leg and flex the top leg to 90°. Using a skin marking pen, draw a line from the greater trochanter to the posterior superior iliac spine and then a second line from the greater trochanter to the sacro-coccygeal joint (or just below the sacral hiatus if the joint is difficult to locate). Draw a third line at 90° from the mid point of the first line to intersect the second line which will usually occur at a point which overlies the sciatic nerve as it leaves the sciatic foramen (Figs 3.14.1, 3.14.2, 3.14.3). Insert an 8 cm 22 G spinal needle at the point of intersection, perpendicular to the skin surface and advance through the gluteal muscles. The needle may strike bone at a depth of 5–6 cm (deeper in a large patient); if so, withdraw the needle slightly and re-direct it in a systematic way until it passes into the sciatic foramen. At this point a peripheral nerve stimulator may be attached to the needle to assist in locating the nerve, or alternatively advance until the patient complains of paraesthesiae in the distribution of the nerve. The nerve is usually found at a depth of 6–8 cm in a patient of medium build. A 10 cm needle may be required in muscular or obese patients. Paraesthesiae are most likely to be elicited in the lateral (peroneal) component of the nerve, i.e. on the lateral aspect of the shin or the dorsum of the foot. A peripheral nerve stimulator will produce dorsiflexion and eversion of the foot. With either technique, providing that the identification is unequivocal, 10–15 ml of high concentration local anaesthetic can be injected without further needle re-positioning to locate the tibial component.

The classical approach is the most proximal of the three described and offers the possibility of the most complete block of all branches of the nerve and is the best route for the insertion of sciatic nerve catheters (p. 164).

Agent	Concn	Volume	Onset	Duration
Bupiv	0.75%	10–15 ml	30 min	12–18 h

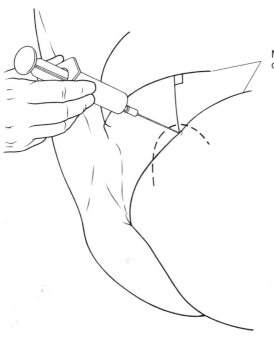

Markings drawn on skin

Fig. 3.14.1
Sciatic nerve block, classical approach

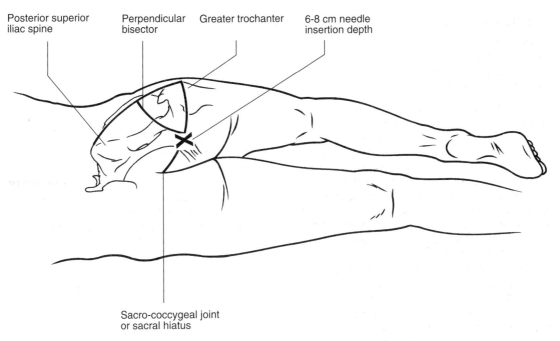

Posterior superior iliac spine

Perpendicular bisector

Greater trochanter

6-8 cm needle insertion depth

Sacro-coccygeal joint or sacral hiatus

Fig. 3.14.2
Sciatic nerve block, posterior view

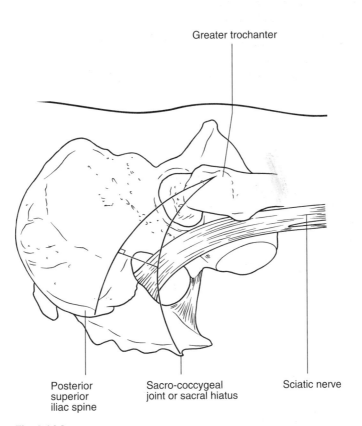

Greater trochanter

Posterior superior iliac spine

Sacro-coccygeal joint or sacral hiatus

Sciatic nerve

Fig. 3.14.3
Sciatic nerve block, landmark details, posterior view

Lithotomy approach

Landmarks
   Greater trochanter
   Ischial tuberosity

Position the patient supine and hold the leg to be blocked in the lithotomy position (with the help of an assistant). It is important that the knee and hip are both flexed to 90° (which limits the use of this approach in patients with trauma or joint disease). Draw a line between the greater trochanter and the ischial tuberosity as in Figure 3.15.3. One centimetre above the midpoint of this line insert an 8 cm 22 G spinal needle perpendicular to the skin (Figs 3.15.1, 3.15.2). The point of insertion usually overlies the groove between the biceps femoris and the semitendinosus muscles and the needle will pass through the intermuscular septum towards the nerve which lies between 5 and 7 cm deep to the skin. If bony contact is made, withdraw the needle slightly and re-angle slightly medially to place the needle tip medial to the lesser trochanter. In this approach the needle may elicit paraesthesiae, or pulse synchronous movement, in either the peroneal or the tibial component of the sciatic nerve as the nerve is being approached in its broadest axis. Compared to peroneal nerve stimulation (refer to classical approach), tibial nerve paraesthesiae occur in the calf or sole of the foot and nerve stimulation produces plantar flexion and inversion of the foot. Following satisfactory location of the nerve inject 8–10 ml of solution.

The lithotomy approach is the easiest to learn as the nerve is at its most superficial and the landmarks are readily identified even in the obese leg. The main drawbacks are the need for assistance in supporting the leg during the procedure and the difficulty in positioning patients with painful joints.

Agent	Concn	Volume	Onset	Duration
Bupiv	0.75%	8–10 ml	30 min	12–18 h

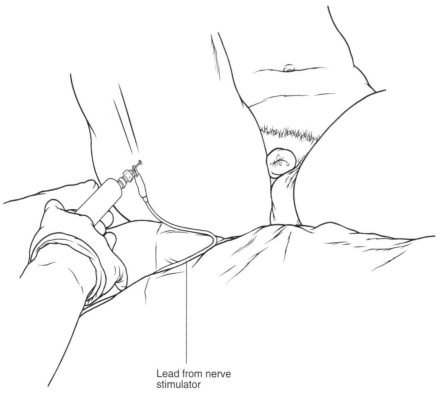

Lead from nerve
stimulator

Fig. 3.15.1
Sciatic nerve block,
lithotomy approach

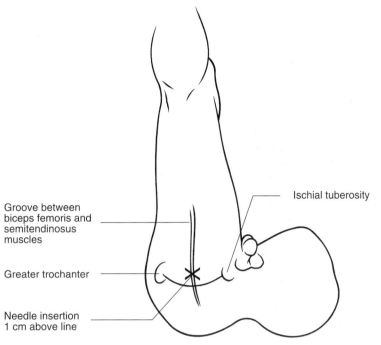

Groove between
biceps femoreen
biceps femoris and
semitendinosus
muscles

Ischial tuberosity

Greater trochanter

Needle insertion
1 cm above line

Fig. 3.15.2
Sciatic nerve block, posterior view

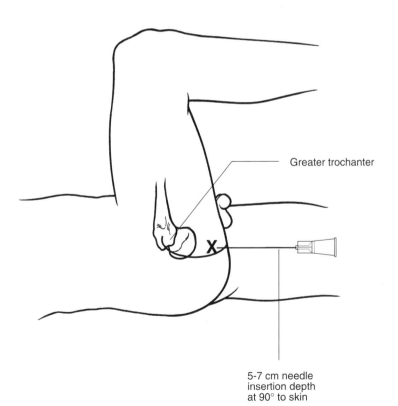

Greater trochanter

5-7 cm needle
insertion depth
at 90° to skin

Fig. 3.15.3
Sciatic nerve block, lateral view

Anterior approach

Landmarks
Inguinal ligament
Greater trochanter

Position the patient supine with the leg slightly abducted, draw a line along the inguinal ligament and divide it into three equal parts marking the junction of the middle and medial thirds. Draw a line from the tuberosity of the greater trochanter parallel to the inguinal ligament across the anterior surface of the thigh. Draw another line at right angles to the inguinal ligament from the junction of the medial and middle thirds to intersect the parallel line (Fig. 3.16.2). Insert a 10 cm insulated short bevel needle at the point of intersection, perpendicular to the skin, in a lateral direction passing medial to the lesser trochanter as shown in Figure 3.16.1, 3.16.3. It is common to hit bone. If this happens, withdraw the needle slightly and re-angle more medially. The sciatic nerve lies just deep to the lesser trochanter in a fascial space behind adductor magnus. Loss of resistance may be felt as the needle enters the space at 8–10 cm depth. After using either paraesthesiae or a nerve stimulator to confirm location (refer to lithotomy approach), inject the solution after negative aspiration.

If a nerve stimulator is used, the depth of this approach and the muscle bulk traversed by the needle makes an insulated needle preferable to an uninsulated needle. The latter causes too much muscle movement artefact and requires a higher power stimulus to locate the nerve. The main benefit of the anterior approach is that the patient does not need to be moved.

Agent	Concn	Volume	Onset	Duration
Bupiv	0.75%	8–15 ml	60 min	12–36 h
Lido	2%	10–20 ml	45 min	8–16 h

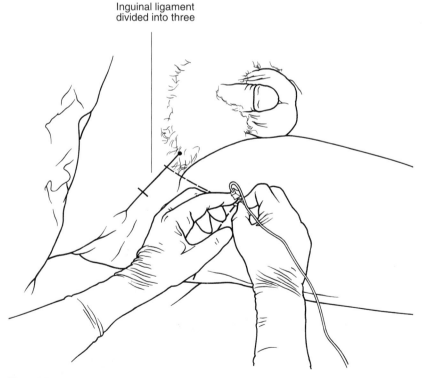

Inguinal ligament
divided into three

Fig. 3.16.1
Sciatic nerve block, anterior approach

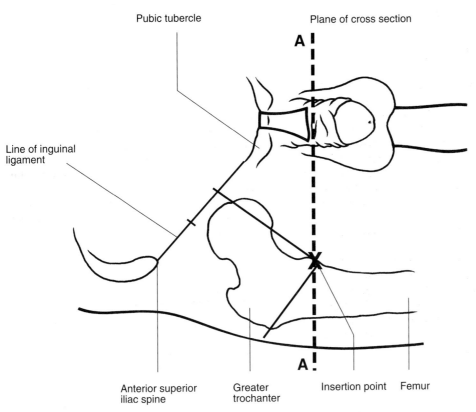

Fig. 3.16.2
Sciatic nerve block, anterior view

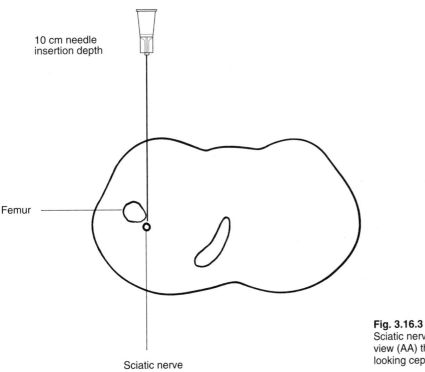

Fig. 3.16.3
Sciatic nerve block, cross sectional view (AA) through needle insertion, looking cephalad

Obturator nerve block

The obturator nerve has the reputation of being difficult to block, with a low success rate and few indications. The classical approach is rather difficult and is uncomfortable for the conscious patient as it requires repeated identification of the bony landmarks which define the obturator canal. However, the 'figure of four' approach is easy to perform and has a high success rate, especially if a peripheral nerve stimulator is used.

Classical approach

Landmarks
   Pubic tubercle
   Superior ramus of pelvis

Position the patient supine with the leg slightly abducted, palpate the pubic tubercle. Raise a skin weal approximately 1–2 cm inferior and 1–2 cm lateral to the tubercle and insert an 8 cm 22 G spinal needle in a cephalad and slightly medial direction, as in Figure 3.17.1, until the lateral aspect of the pubis is contacted. Withdraw the needle slightly and redirect it laterally towards the anterior superior iliac spine retaining the same angle to the skin (Fig. 3.17.2). Usually the needle contacts the superior pubic ramus just above the obturator canal, although the needle may directly enter the canal. If the ramus is identified, re-angle the needle by raising the hub and directing it inferiorly until the obturator canal is entered (this will be felt as a slight resistance followed by a 'give' when the needle penetrates the obturator membrane).

Limited and variable cutaneous innervation means that paraesthesiae may not be elicited in the conscious patient and a peripheral nerve stimulator will give a more accurate location by producing pulse synchronous movement of the adductor muscles. Inject the solution after aspiration.

Agent	Concn	Volume	Onset	Duration
Bupiv	0.5%	10 ml	20 min	6–12 h
Bupiv	0.75%	5–7 ml	15 min	12–18 h

Finger palpating
pubic tubercle

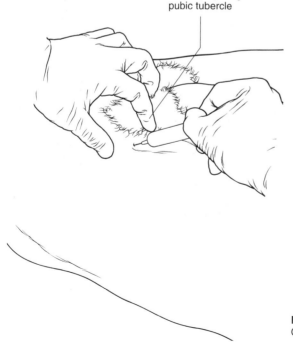

Fig. 3.17.1
Obturator nerve block, classical approach

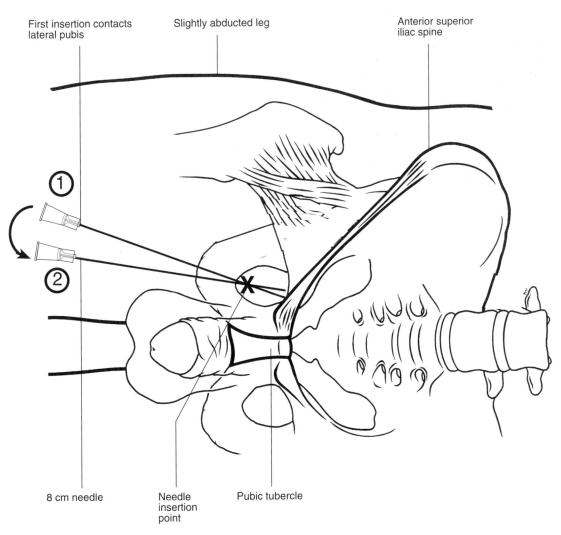

First insertion contacts lateral pubis

Slightly abducted leg

Anterior superior iliac spine

8 cm needle

Needle insertion point

Pubic tubercle

Fig. 3.17.2
Obturator nerve block, anterior view

'Figure of four' approach

Landmarks
  Insertion of the adductor muscle tendons

Position the patient supine and place the leg in the 'figure of four' position. Identify the insertion of the adductor magnus and the adductor brevis muscles into the pubis. Raise a skin weal over the gap between the tendons about 1 cm inferior to the pubis (Fig. 3.18.1). Insert an 8 cm spinal needle in the horizontal plane aiming towards the anterior superior iliac spine. At a depth of approximately 5 cm, the resistance of the obturator membrane will be felt and a slight 'pop' may also occur (Figs 3.18.2, 3.18.3). At this point, after aspiration, inject 5 ml of solution. Alternatively a peripheral nerve stimulator may be used to confirm accurate placement of the needle prior to injection when pulse synchronous contraction of the adductor muscles will be seen. The needle will directly enter the foramen in the majority of cases but if the bony boundaries of the foramen are encountered, the needle should be withdrawn slightly and re-directed appropriately.

The advantage of the 'figure of four' approach is that needle insertion is in a single, consistent direction which places the needle tip close to the division of the nerve into its two branches, an important factor in achieving complete block of the motor and cutaneous distribution.

Agent	Concn	Volume	Onset	Duration
Bupiv	0.5%	10–15 ml	20 min	6–12 h
Bupiv	0.75%	5–7 ml	15 min	12–18 h

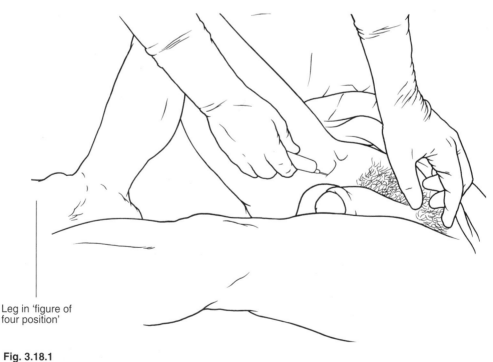

Leg in 'figure of four position'

Fig. 3.18.1
Obturator nerve block, 'figure of four' position

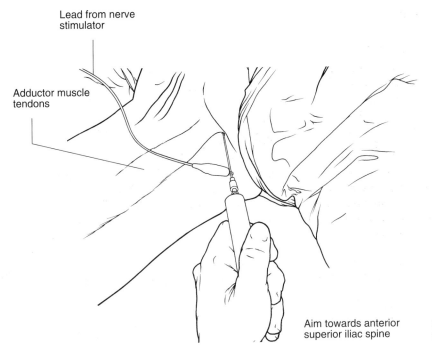

Lead from nerve
stimulator

Adductor muscle
tendons

Aim towards anterior
superior iliac spine

Fig. 3.18.2
Obturator nerve block

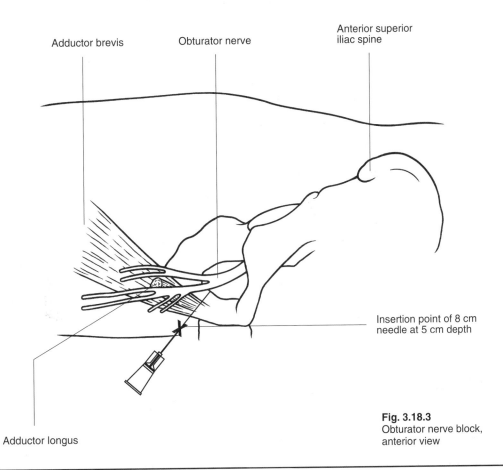

Adductor brevis

Obturator nerve

Anterior superior
iliac spine

Insertion point of 8 cm
needle at 5 cm depth

Adductor longus

Fig. 3.18.3
Obturator nerve block,
anterior view

Technique **89**

Lumbar plexus block

The standard proximal approach to the lumbar plexus is paravertebral and the original descriptions are based on multiple injections – one at each lumbar transverse process. More recently, new techniques have been described which only require a single needle insertion at either the L2, 3 or L3, 4 interspaces.

Controversy. There is controversy about the particular mode of action of these techniques, particularly where large volumes of local anaesthetic are used because it is possible for the local anaesthetic to flow into the epidural space and produce most of its effects as an epidural block.

Lumbar paravertebral block

Landmarks
  Spinous processes of lumbar spine

Place the patient prone over a pillow placed under the abdomen. Identify the spinous processes. Mark a point 3–4 cm lateral to the cephalad edge of the third lumbar spine and insert an 8 cm 22 G spinal needle perpendicular to the skin until the transverse process is contacted, as in Figure 3.19.1. This usually occurs at a depth of 4–5 cm, at which point the needle is withdrawn slightly and re-angled both cephalad and medially (approximately 25–30° to the midline). Advance the needle slowly so that it just passes cephalad to the proximal edge of the transverse process and 2–3 cm deep to the transverse process. Paraesthesiae will be elicited in the L2 nerve root. Inject 20–30 ml of solution after careful aspiration to ensure that cerebrospinal fluid or blood are not present. A dilute solution will suffice because the local anaesthetic is applied directly to the nerve roots in large volume.

Agent	Concn	Volume	Onset	Duration
Bupiv	0.25%	20–30 ml	45 min	4 h

Lumbar plexus block

Landmarks
  Spinous processes of lumbar spine

The procedure is identical to the paravertebral technique except that having contacted the transverse process, the needle should be withdrawn and re-angled cephalad, but not medially (Figs 3.19.2, 3.19.3). Keep to a plane parallel to the midline and advance about 2 cm beyond the transverse process. At this point, entry into the psoas compartment can be confirmed by loss of resistance to air from an attached syringe. After negative aspiration for blood, inject 15–20 ml of solution.

The psoas compartment block is a particular description of a single needle insertion at L4, 5 and may just be a modification of the technique described above.

Agent	Concn	Volume	Onset	Duration
Bupiv	0.25%	20–30 ml	20 min	3–5 h
Bupiv	0.5%	15–20 ml	20 min	4–8 h

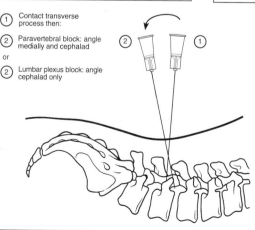

① Contact transverse process then:

② Paravertebral block: angle medially and cephalad

or

② Lumbar plexus block: angle cephalad only

Fig. 3.19.1
Lumbar plexus block, lateral view

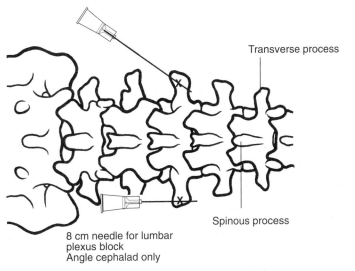

8 cm needle for paravertebral block
Angle medially and cephalad

Transverse process

Spinous process

8 cm needle for lumbar plexus block
Angle cephalad only

Fig. 3.19.2
Lumbar plexus block, posterior view

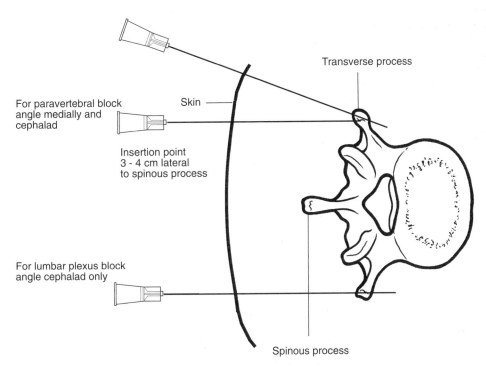

Transverse process

For paravertebral block angle medially and cephalad

Skin

Insertion point
3 - 4 cm lateral to spinous process

For lumbar plexus block angle cephalad only

Spinous process

Fig. 3.19.3
Lumbar plexus block, cross sectional view

Lateral cutaneous nerve of thigh block

Landmarks
   Anterior superior iliac spine
   Inguinal ligament
   Fascia lata

Position the patient supine and palpate the anterior superior iliac spine to define the insertion of the inguinal ligament. Insert a 3.5 cm short bevelled needle 2–3 cm below the spine and 2–3 cm medial, as in Figure 3.20.1. A few millimetres below the surface, the fascia lata will be felt as a definite resistance to the needle and if the needle is moved slightly each way in the horizontal plane, the fascia can be 'scratched'. Advance the needle through the fascia with a definite 'pop' and inject 10 ml of solution immediately deep to the fascia (Fig. 3.20.2).

The nerve can also be blocked by an approach above the inguinal ligament but the end point is more difficult to identify and this is therefore not recommended.

Agent	Concn	Volume	Onset	Duration
Bupiv	0.5%	10 ml	20 min	4–6 h

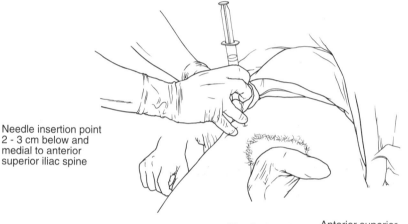

Needle insertion point 2 - 3 cm below and medial to anterior superior iliac spine

Fig. 3.20.1
Lateral cutaneous nerve of thigh block

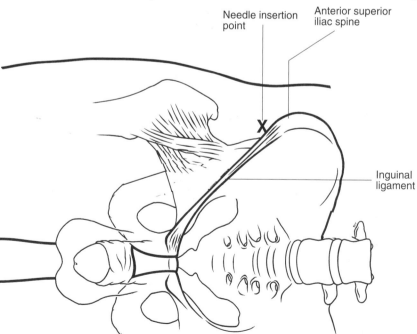

Needle insertion point

Anterior superior iliac spine

Inguinal ligament

Fig. 3.20.2
Lateral cutaneous nerve, anterior view

Iliac crest block

The subcostal nerve (T12) can be difficult to block at the level of the 12th rib in the obese or immobile patient. For hip surgery it is more easily approached via the iliac crest.

Landmarks
  Anterior superior iliac spine (ASIS)
  Iliac crest

Make a subcutaneous injection of solution from the ASIS posteriorly along the iliac crest using an 8 cm 22 G spinal needle (Fig. 3.21.1).

Agent	Concn	Volume	Onset	Duration
Bupiv	0.5%	10 ml	20 min	8 h
Prilo	1%	10 ml	10 min	4 h

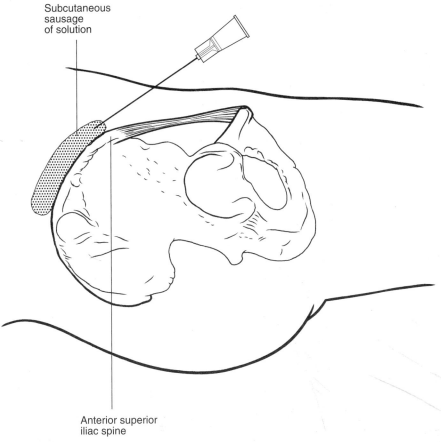

Subcutaneous
sausage
of solution

Anterior superior
iliac spine

Fig. 3.21.1
Iliac crest block, lateral view

Penile block

Landmarks
  Symphysis pubis

Position the patient supine and stand on the right. Palpate the distal edge of the symphysis pubis with the index finger of the left hand and introduce a 21 G needle as in Figure 3.22.2, just distal to the index finger. Advance the needle until it contacts the distal leading edge of the pubis at which point it should have passed through the deep 'Buck's' fascia of the penis (Fig. 3.22.1). Inject 5–7 ml of solution after careful negative aspiration for blood.

> Note. On no account should solutions contain any vasoconstrictor.

Provided that the needle is in the correct plane there is no need to reposition or make a second injection as both dorsal nerves are reliably blocked with this approach. Complete the block by making a subcutaneous injection of 3–5 ml of solution across the root of the penis. Start 2 cm lateral to the midline and inject continuously as the needle is advanced across the median raphe, finishing 2 cm beyond it on the other side (Fig 3.22.3). It is important to keep the needle subcutaneous in the midline because the urethra is very superficial at the base of the penis.

Agent	Concn	Volume	Onset	Duration
Bupiv	0.5%	10 ml	10 min	8 h

Inferior border
pubic symphysis

Artery

Nerve

Finger

Buck's fascia

Fig. 3.22.1
Penile block, coronal section

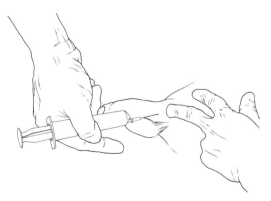

Fig. 3.22.2
Penile block

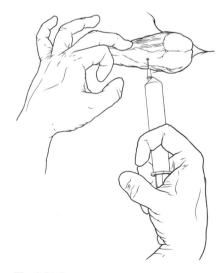

Fig. 3.22.3
Penile block, completion

Scrotal infiltration

Unilateral or bilateral inguinal canal blocks need to be supplemented by scrotal infiltration to achieve complete analgesia of the testes. Make the injection in the median raphe if surgery involves both testes. For unilateral surgery infiltrate over the anterior aspect of the relevant side of the scrotum. The injection should be made in consultation with the surgeon to ensure that it covers the site of incision. If a vasoconstrictor is added to solution, it will aid haemostasis and indicate to the surgeon where to incise (Figs 3.23.1, 3.23.2).

Agent	Concn	Volume	Onset	Duration
Bupiv + adren	0.5%	10 ml	5 min	8 h

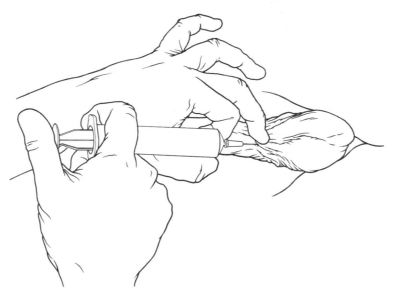

Fig. 3.23.1
Scrotal infiltration

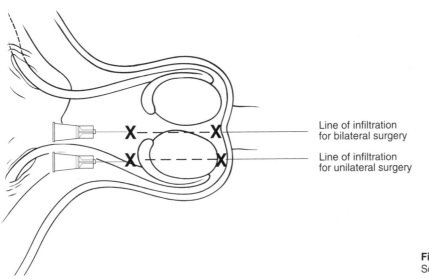

Line of infiltration
for bilateral surgery

Line of infiltration
for unilateral surgery

Fig. 3.23.2
Scrotal infiltration, details

Inguinal field block

The technique requires discrete blockade of three nerves, the ilioinguinal, the iliohypogastric and the genitofemoral. In addition, subcutaneous infiltration of the abdominal wall is necessary to block overlapping nerve fibres from adjacent dermatomes.

Landmarks
Anterior superior iliac spine (ASIS)
Pubic tubercle

Position the patient supine and palpate the ASIS. Insert a 22 G short bevel needle perpendicularly at a point 2 cm medial and inferior to the ASIS (Fig. 3.24.1). Advance the needle carefully through the subcutaneous tissues until resistance indicates that the aponeurosis of the external oblique muscle has been reached. If the needle is now moved from side to side, it will move freely in the subcutaneous tissues and scratch on the aponeurosis. Further advancement of the needle will produce a distinct 'pop' as it penetrates the tough fascia and side-to-side movement of the needle is no longer possible. The iliohypogastric nerve lies immediately deep to the aponeurosis and an injection of 5–7 ml of solution is sufficient to block it at this point. Now advance the needle a further 1–2 cm through the softer resistance of the internal oblique muscle and inject a further 5–7 ml of solution to block the ilioinguinal nerve which is lying deep to the muscle before it penetrates the internal oblique to gain entry to the inguinal canal (Fig. 3.24.2).

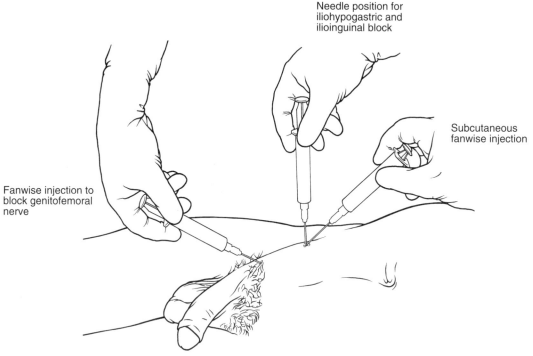

Needle position for iliohypogastric and ilioinguinal block

Subcutaneous fanwise injection

Fanwise injection to block genitofemoral nerve

Fig. 3.24.1
Inguinal field block

After the deep injection is complete, withdraw the needle to the skin and re-direct to inject a further 10 ml of solution subcutaneously in a fanwise distribution so that any cutaneous innervation from the subcostal nerve is blocked. An alternative technique involves a single injection of 15–20 ml just deep to the aponeurosis which should block both the iliohypogastric at the point of injection and the ilioinguinal distally as it emerges through the internal oblique muscle into the same plane as the iliohypogastric. The genitofemoral nerve is most reliably blocked by the inguinal canal block (pp. 98–99). If this is not possible due to an irreducible hernia or other anatomical abnormality, the lower end of the field block will require an injection of 10 ml of solution fanwise from the pubic tubercle towards the external inguinal ring and then towards the midline. This will block the fibres of genitofemoral and ilioinguinal as they emerge from the inguinal canal and also block any fibres which cross the midline. Using up to 30 ml of concentrated local anaesthetic gives post-operative analgesia of up to 12 hours. In the conscious patient it is necessary to use a larger volume of more dilute local anaesthetic because the surgeon may have to supplement the block with direct injection into some of the deeper structures.

Agent	Concn	Volume	Onset	Duration
Bupiv + adren	0.5%	30 ml	10 min	12 h
Bupiv + adren	0.25%	40 ml	20 min	6 h

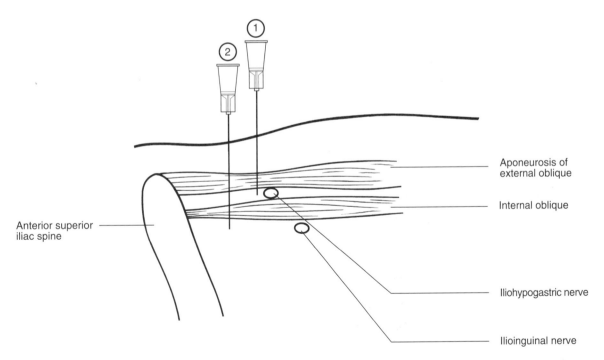

Fig. 3.24.2
Iliohypogastric (1) and ilioinguinal (2) nerve blocks, cross section view

Anterior superior iliac spine

Aponeurosis of external oblique

Internal oblique

Iliohypogastric nerve

Ilioinguinal nerve

Inguinal canal block

Inguinal canal block is indicated to supplement inguinal field block and also to anaesthetise the scrotal contents for a variety of urological operations. It is important to ensure that the inguinal canal contains only its normal structures (the spermatic cord and the ilioinguinal nerve) prior to performing this technique.

Landmarks
    Anterior superior iliac spine (ASIS)
    Pubic tubercle
    External inguinal ring

Palpate the inguinal ligament between the ASIS and the pubic tubercle. Approximately 1 cm above its midpoint, the deep inguinal ring can be palpated as a 'U' shaped depression (Fig. 3.25.1). In the obese patient or where previous surgery has made the landmarks difficult to palpate, the ring may be difficult to feel. In such cases, the skin of the scrotum can be invaginated with a finger and the external and deep rings identified. Having confirmed that the inguinal canal contains no hernial contents, place the index finger of the left hand on the deep ring to identify its position and insert a short bevel needle parallel to the inguinal ligament about 1 cm distal to the index finger, at 45° to the skin and aimed towards the deep ring (Fig. 3.25.2). There is usually a distinct 'pop' as the needle penetrates the external oblique aponeurosis and enters the inguinal canal. Hold the needle firmly in position and inject 5 ml of solution. The inguinal canal is usually 1–2 cm deep to the surface. It is important not to advance the needle too far once the canal has been entered because the femoral vessels and the femoral nerve lie immediately deep to the canal. If this block is used as part of an inguinal field block, then after injecting 5 ml into the canal, the needle can be withdrawn to the skin and re-directed to inject a further 5–10 ml subcutaneously to complete the technique.

Agent	Concn	Volume	Onset	Duration
Bupiv	0.5%	5 ml	10 min	8 h

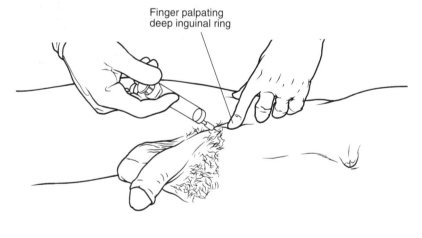

Finger palpating
deep inguinal ring

Fig. 3.25.1
Inguinal canal block

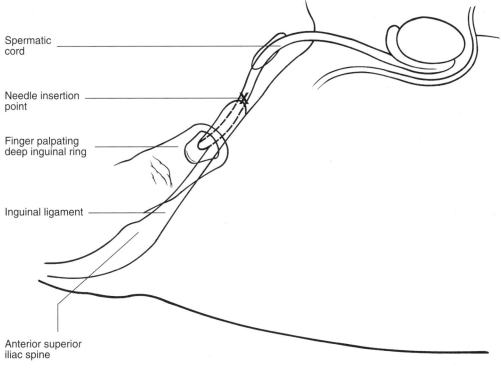

Spermatic
cord

Needle insertion
point

Finger palpating
deep inguinal ring

Inguinal ligament

Anterior superior
iliac spine

Fig. 3.25.2
Inguinal canal block, anterior view

Intercostal nerve block

Landmarks
  Angle of each rib
  Mid axillary line

The position of the patient will depend on whether the patient is anaesthetised or conscious and whether they are to receive unilateral or bilateral blockade. For unilateral blocks, place the patient in the lateral position as in Figure 3.26.1, with the side to be blocked uppermost. For bilateral intercostal blocks, the patient should either be in the prone position or, if conscious, sat upright on the edge of the bed leaning forward on a table for support.

The ribs are easily palpated in patients of normal or thin build but in the obese patient they can be very difficult to define and this may be a relative contraindication to the technique. The same approach is used for each rib and begins with palpating the rib to identify the rib angle which is usually found 8 cm lateral to the vertebral spine. The exact point of insertion of the needle is not crucial as long as it is posterior to the mid axillary line, where the lateral cutaneous branch of each intercostal nerve arises.

It is customary to count the ribs upwards from the 12th rib, which is easy to identify due to its short length. Having reliably identified each rib, raise a skin bleb of local anaesthetic with a 25 G needle and infiltrate down to the periosteum. Repeat for each intended level. Intercostal nerve blocks require multiple injections and many patients find them painful unless the anaesthetist is very gentle and sedation may be necessary. It may also be helpful to mark the sites of injection with a skin marker because this lessens the likelihood of inadvertently injecting the same intercostal space twice.

Make the skin blebs at the inferior edge of the ribs so that when the main injection is made, the skin can be gently pulled cephalad with the index finger of the left hand until the point of insertion lies over the body of the rib. Insert a 22 G, 3 cm short bevel needle perpendicular to the skin until contact is made with the rib periosteum at which point support the needle firmly between thumb and index finger and 'walk' the needle off the inferior edge of the rib as the skin which was stretched over the rib returns to its normal position. When the needle reaches the inferior edge of the rib, cautiously advance 3–4 mm under the firm control of the left hand, which should be braced against the patient's back. With short bevelled needles, a 'pop' may be felt as the needle penetrates the external intercostal muscle at its origin on the intercostal groove. Inject 3–4 ml of solution (Fig. 3.26.2). As the thoracic nerves have both motor and sensory fibres, it is possible to use a nerve stimulator to identify each intercostal nerve by observing abdominal (not intercostal) muscle movement. In practice, however, nerve stimulators are rarely necessary for this procedure.

Controversy. It is uncertain as to whether it is necessary to block each intercostal nerve to achieve a clinically effective block. Single space injections of a large volume have been described which may in effect be similar to a thoracic paravertebral injection as the intercostal space is a continuation of the paravertebral space. Indwelling intercostal space catheters have also been described for long term analgesia thus avoiding the need for repeated injections.

If bilateral blocks are performed, large volumes of local anaesthetic solution will be needed and because the intercostal spaces are very vascular there is a risk of rapid absorption. It is thus very important to avoid intravascular injection and to observe the patient closely for signs of early toxicity

Pneumothorax is a major complication, the risk of which decreases with the experience of the practitioner. Nevertheless, the higher the number of spaces to be blocked, the greater the risk becomes.

For unilateral blocks, the risk to the patient is small as any pneumothorax is usually minor. Nitrous oxide administration may, however, increase the size of any pneumothorax

Agent	Concn	Volume	Onset	Duration
Bupiv	0.5%	3–4 ml	10 min	4 h

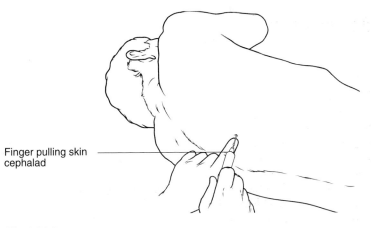

Fig. 3.26.1
Intercostal nerve block

Finger pulling skin cephalad

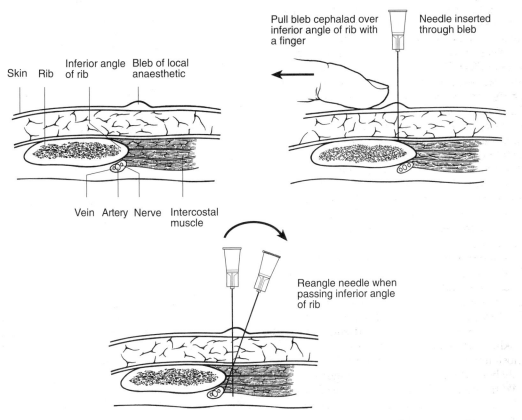

Skin   Rib   Inferior angle of rib   Bleb of local anaesthetic

Vein   Artery   Nerve   Intercostal muscle

Pull bleb cephalad over inferior angle of rib with a finger

Needle inserted through bleb

Reangle needle when passing inferior angle of rib

Fig. 3.26.2
Intercostal nerve block, cross sectional views

Thoracic paravertebral block

Used more commonly in the diagnosis and treatment of chronic pain than for post-operative pain relief, thoracic paravertebral block has a role in patients requiring unilateral analgesia (e.g. fractured ribs, thoracotomy or nephrectomy) in whom a thoracic epidural is inappropriate.

Landmarks

Thoracic vertebral spinous processes

Position the patient prone or in the lateral position. Identify the spinous process of the appropriate thoracic vertebra, bearing in mind that because of the acute angulation of the thoracic spines, the spinous process of the vertebra above the nerve to be blocked must be used. At a point 3 cm lateral to the cephalad edge of the spinous process, insert an 8 cm spinal needle as in Figure 3.27.1, and advance until the transverse process is struck at a depth of 3–4 cm. Withdraw slightly, and re-angle cephalad so that the needle tip just 'walks off' the cephalad edge of the transverse process and advance a further 2 cm (Figs 3.27.2, 3.27.3). It is important that the needle is not directed medially as this may result in an epidural placement or inadvertent puncture of the dural cuff of the thoracic nerve. If the needle is too lateral, it may produce an intercostal block or enter the pleural cavity. As the needle is advanced beyond the transverse process, it passes through the costotransverse ligament and a change in tissue resistance can be felt as it enters the looser fatty tissue of the paravertebral space. Loss of resistance to saline can be used to confirm the needle position and in the conscious patient, paraesthesiae may occur in the distribution of the nerve. A peripheral nerve stimulator can also be used to confirm accurate needle placement as pulse synchronous movement of the rectus muscle should be visible. Careful aspiration to ensure that no CSF or blood is obtained should be followed by slow injection of the solution. The spread of local anaesthetic in the paravertebral space is very variable. As little as 5 ml may affect 1–6 dermatomes and can produce bilateral effects from penetration of the epidural space. On average 3–4 dermatomes are blocked by injecting 5 ml at one level; if a more extensive spread is required, the procedure can be repeated at another space, or a catheter can be inserted (p. 163). Sequential doses may be given until the desired spread is achieved.

Complications

Pneumothorax (up to 20% incidence), intradural injection and epidural spread.

Agent	Concn	Volume	Onset	Duration
Bupiv	0.5%	5 ml	10 min	4 h

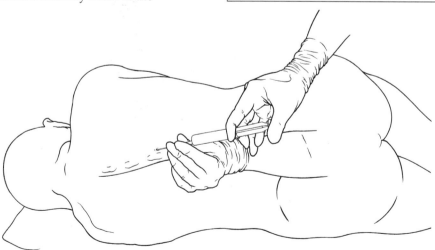

Fig. 3.27.1
Thoracic paravertebral block

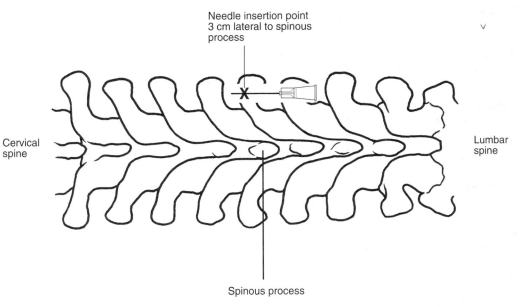

Needle insertion point
3 cm lateral to spinous
process

Cervical
spine

Lumbar
spine

Spinous process

Fig. 3.27.2
Paravertebral block, posterior view

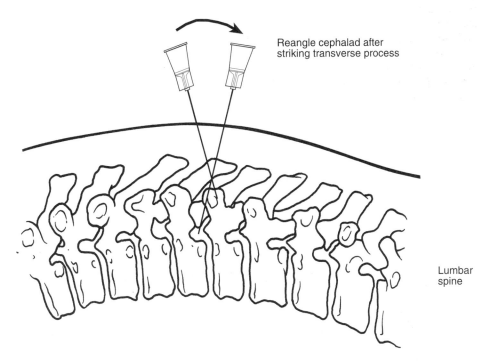

Reangle cephalad after
striking transverse process

Cervical
spine

Lumbar
spine

Fig. 3.27.3
Paravertebral block, lateral view

Interpleural block

Landmarks
  Angle of the 6th rib

Position the patient laterally as for intercostal block and identify the 6th (or 7th) rib (Fig. 3.28.1). The risk of causing a clinically significant pneumothorax is always present because the intention is to deliberately enter the pleural cavity. This may result from air being entrained through the needle or direct lung damage. A number of techniques have been described, each claiming to reduce the risk of pneumothorax. The use of a simple one-way or self-sealing valve with a side arm (Arrow Catheter Sheath Adaptor SV 07000) completely excludes the entry of air into the pleural cavity (Scott 1991) (Fig. 3.28.3). In the anaesthetised patient, introduce a 16 G Tuohy needle at the angle of the rib and aim at 45° towards the upper edge of the rib, thus avoiding the intercostal neurovascular bundle (Fig. 3.28.2). Connect the side arm of the one-way valve to a giving set primed with 500 ml of normal saline.

Attach the valve to the needle and open the roller clamp of the giving set. Walk the needle off the upper border of the rib and advance into the pleural cavity, at which point there will be a loss of resistance and the saline will run freely into the space. Hold the needle firmly between thumb and forefinger of the left hand, to prevent further advancement towards the lung and insert the epidural catheter through the needle and valve into the pleural cavity until 8 cm lies within the space. Remove the needle and secure the catheter with an airtight dressing. The insertion of the needle should be carried out with the lung at end expiration to reduce the risk of damage. Inject 20 ml of solution through the catheter. Head down tilt will improve upper thoracic dermatomal anaesthesia but may also produce Horner's syndrome.

Agent	Concn	Volume	Onset	Duration
Bupiv	0.5%	20 ml	10 min	8 h

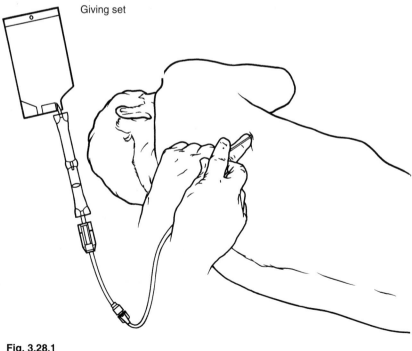

Giving set

Fig. 3.28.1
Interpleural block

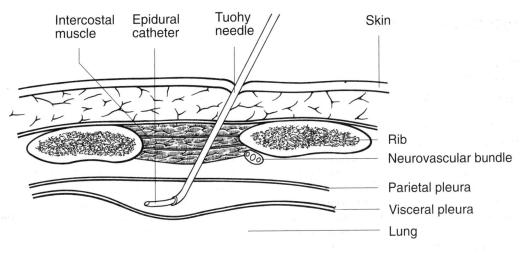

Fig. 3.28.2
Interpleural block, cross section view

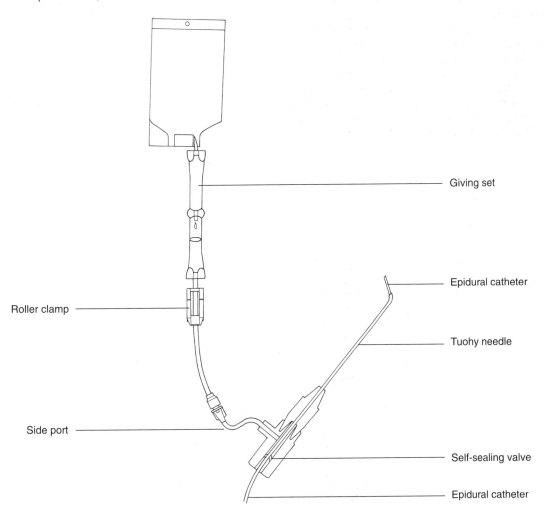

Fig. 3.28.3
Interpleural block, needle connections

Brachial plexus block

Blockade of the brachial plexus is the most frequently performed major peripheral nerve block. Over 40 techniques are described in the literature, falling into four groups: interscalene, supraclavicular, axillary and infraclavicular. The infraclavicular approach is the least popular as it requires a peripheral nerve stimulator and 8 cm insulated needles which have to traverse the pectoralis muscles, making the approach uncomfortable for conscious patients.

General considerations

No one technique is clearly better than the others as all have different benefits and complications. The axillary approach is the easiest technique to learn and has the lowest incidence of complications. The key to success is the reliable entry of the fascial sheath investing the plexus because it is possible to influence the spread of solution by adjusting the volume of the injection and by using digital pressure to achieve the required area of anaesthesia for the proposed surgery on the arm. Winnie's monograph on brachial plexus blockade (1983), describes a detailed investigation of the relationships between the site of injection, the volume of injection and the use of digital pressure. The use of 40 ml of solution, with appropriate digital pressure, in a healthy male adult produces satisfactory spread whichever approach is used. Patient positions are shown in Figures 3.29.1, 3.29.2.

Peripheral nerve blocks

In the event that a brachial plexus block is inadequate for surgery, the five terminal nerves (pp. 118–125) can be blocked singly or in combination to reinforce the plexus block.

Equipment

The concept of the 'immobile needle' is important. By using a 10–20 cm extension tube, the needle can be isolated from the movements of the syringe during aspiration and injection or during changing of syringes. The needle must be short bevelled to decrease the risk of nerve damage and to increase the feel of resistance as the needle encounters the fascia. A peripheral nerve stimulator is a useful aid to confirm accurate positioning of the needle tip, especially for the more proximal approaches.

Complications

Serious complications can occur with any of the approaches to the brachial plexus. Some complications are common to all regional anaesthetic techniques but others are specific to the different approaches – see Table 3.1.

Table 3.1 Complications of brachial plexus block

	Axillary	Supraclavicular	Interscalene	Comments
vertebral artery injection	–	+/–	++	rare but lethal
subarachnoid/epidural injection	–	+	++	rare but dangerous
phrenic nerve palsy	+/–	++	+++	36–90% incidence usually asymptomatic
recurrent laryngeal nerve palsy	–	+	+	1.5–6% incidence
stellate ganglion block	+	++	+++	50–90% incidence
pneumothorax	+/–	+++	+	0.6–25% incidence usually asymptomatic

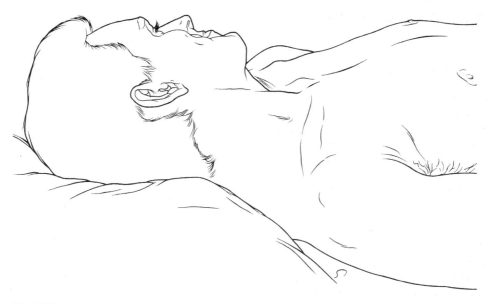

Fig. 3.29.1
Patient position for interscalene and supraclavicular block

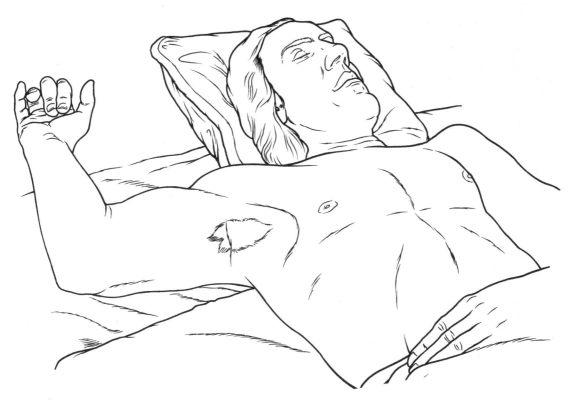

Fig. 3.29.2
Patient position for axillary block

Supraclavicular approach (subclavian perivascular technique)

Landmarks
Cricoid cartilage
Posterior border of sternomastoid interscalene groove
Clavicle
Pulsation of subclavian artery

Position the patient supine with a small pillow under the head and neck, turning the head slightly away from the side to be blocked. Push the shoulder downwards to depress the clavicle. A line drawn laterally from the cricoid cartilage will cross the sternomastoid at its mid point (often meeting the external jugular vein at the posterior border of the sternomastoid muscle). If the muscle is difficult to palpate, it may be put under tension by instructing the patient to raise their head whilst keeping it turned to the side. The interscalene groove should be located behind the mid point of the posterior border of the muscle. To confirm this position, the middle and anterior interscalene muscles can be highlighted by asking the patient to inspire vigorously or 'sniff'. The interscalene groove may then be followed distally towards the clavicle. In some patients, the trunks of the plexus can be palpated in the groove by rolling the finger gently from side to side; this may produce paraesthesiae. Approximately 1 cm above the midpoint of the clavicle, the pulsation of the subclavian artery can be felt in the interscalene groove. Stand to the side of the patient. On the right side, palpate the interscalene groove with the left index finger and insert the needle with the right hand, reversing the hands for the opposite approach (Fig. 3.30.1). The ideal position for needle insertion is just above the pulsation of the subclavian artery, although a more medial and proximal point is adequate as long as the groove is palpated with certainty. After injecting an intradermal weal of local anaesthetic, insert a 22 G short bevel 3.5 cm needle caudally in the horizontal plane, parallel to the neck and it will enter the fascial sheath 1–2 cm deep to the skin. Marked resistance will give way to a 'pop' as the fascia is pierced and paraesthesiae may

occur (Fig. 3.30.2). It is important to ascertain from the patient that the 'pins and needles' are in an appropriate distribution of the plexus (paraesthesiae around the shoulder should not be relied upon). Paraesthesiae most commonly occur in the distribution of the superior trunk because of the vertical arrangement of the nerve trunks. A peripheral nerve stimulator can be used to confirm needle placement.

Once paraesthesiae are elicited it is not necessary to hunt for other trunks. Hold the needle firmly in position and carefully aspirate to exclude intravascular placement, then make the injection. If arterial blood is aspirated, carefully withdraw the needle until blood ceases to flow (because the subclavian artery is within the sheath, the needle will still be in the brachial plexus) and then inject. Solution should flow without resistance. High resistance or pain on injection may indicate intraneural injection and the needle must be repositioned at once.

Up to 40 ml of solution can be used depending on the mass of the patient and the desired extent of the block. When using large volumes the sheath may be felt to distend during the injection; this is normal and is easily distinguished from the subcutaneous swelling of an extra fascial injection. To encourage proximal spread (and thus simulate an interscalene block) digital pressure distal to the needle insertion point may be used during the latter part of the injection. Similarly, digital pressure proximal to the needle insertion may help to encourage distal spread.

Agent	Concn	Volume	Onset	Duration
Bupiv	0.5%	25–40 ml	40 min	4–12 h
Prilo	2%	25–40 ml	20 min	3–5 h

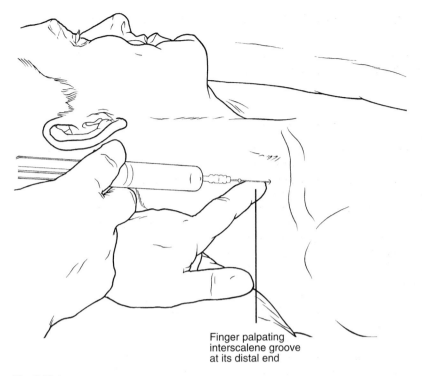

Finger palpating
interscalene groove
at its distal end

Fig. 3.30.1
Brachial plexus block, supraclavicular block

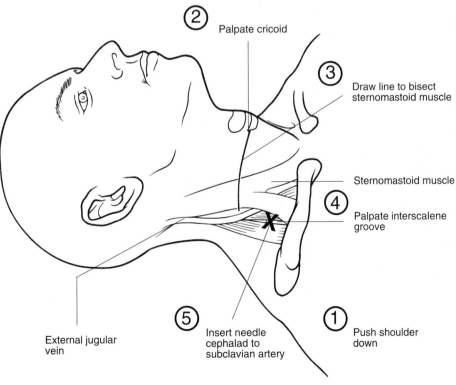

② Palpate cricoid

③ Draw line to bisect
sternomastoid muscle

Sternomastoid muscle

④ Palpate interscalene
groove

X

External jugular
vein

⑤ Insert needle
cephalad to
subclavian artery

① Push shoulder
down

Fig. 3.30.2
Supraclavicular block, lateral view

Interscalene approach

Landmarks
Cricoid cartilage
Posterior border sternomastoid muscle
Interscalene groove

Position the patient supine with a small pillow under the head and neck and the head turned slightly away from the side to be blocked. Push the shoulder downwards to depress the clavicle. A line drawn lateral from the cricoid cartilage will cross the sternomastoid at its midpoint. If the muscle is difficult to palpate, the patient can put it under tension by raising the head whilst keeping it turned to the side. Locate the interscalene groove behind the midpoint of the posterior border of the sternomastoid muscle with a palpating finger, as in Figure 3.31.1. This may be confirmed by asking the patient to inspire vigorously or 'sniff' which will throw the anterior and middle scalene muscles into relief. Stand at the side of the patient and after locating the interscalene groove, raise an intradermal weal at the point of needle insertion which is usually at the level of the cricoid cartilage. Insert a 22 G 3.5 cm short bevel needle aiming fractionally dorsal to the horizontal plane. The fascial sheath will usually be entered with a 'pop' between 1 and 2.5 cm deep to the skin. Advance the needle slowly (Figs 3.31.2, 3.31.3) until paraesthesiae are elicited in the distribution of the arm or hand (not the shoulder or neck). A peripheral nerve stimulator can be used to confirm needle placement. Careful aspiration is necessary to detect inadvertent entry into the vertebral artery or the dural cuff of a cervical nerve after which slow injection should be made with repeated aspiration. Digital pressure proximal to the needle will encourage caudal spread.

Agent	Concn	Volume	Onset	Duration
Bupiv	0.5%	20 ml	40 min	4–12 h
Prilo	2%	20 ml	20 min	4–6 h

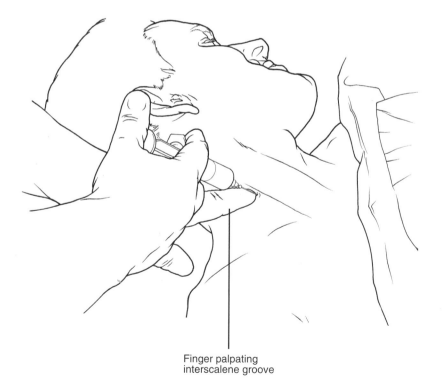

Finger palpating
interscalene groove

Fig. 3.31.1
Brachial plexus block, interscalene approach

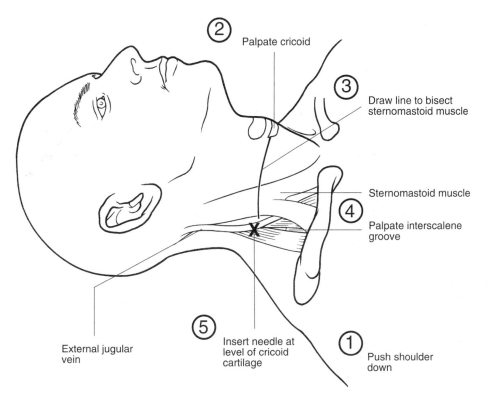

② Palpate cricoid

③ Draw line to bisect sternomastoid muscle

Sternomastoid muscle

④ Palpate interscalene groove

External jugular vein

⑤ Insert needle at level of cricoid cartilage

① Push shoulder down

Fig. 3.31.2
Interscalene block, lateral view

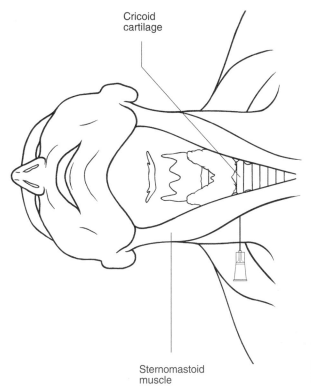

Cricoid cartilage

Sternomastoid muscle

Fig. 3.31.3
Interscalene block, anterior view

Axillary approach

Landmarks
    Axillary artery pulsation
    Lateral border of pectoralis major

Position the patient supine with the arm to be blocked abducted to 90° at the shoulder and the elbow flexed to 90° as in Figure 3.32.1. Do not over abduct the arm because the pulsation of the artery may be diminished by pressure from the head of the humerus.

Palpate the pulsation of the axillary artery at the level of the lateral border of the pectoralis major and fix the artery with the palpating finger (Fig. 3.32.2). Insert a 3.5 cm 22 G short bevel needle through an intradermal skin weal, just superior to the artery until the resistance of the fascial sheath is felt and a 'pop' indicates that the needle has entered the sheath (Fig. 3.32.3). Paraesthesiae indicate correct needle placement and a peripheral nerve stimulator can be used to confirm this. After negative aspiration, inject local anaesthetic solution using digital pressure distal to the needle to encourage proximal spread. When injection is complete, maintain the digital pressure whilst the arm is adducted so that the humoral head no longer obstructs the upward flow of solution. If blood is aspirated, this indicates intra-arterial needle placement. In this case, the needle can either be withdrawn and repositioned within the sheath or it may be deliberately advanced further until no more blood can be aspirated and the injection made deep to the artery (the transarterial technique).

The musculocutaneous nerve may not be blocked adequately by the axillary approach. If necessary, the nerve can be blocked separately after completion of the axillary injection by withdrawing the needle from the sheath and redirecting it at 90° to the skin and superior to the artery (Fig. 3.32.3). Advance the needle into the coracobrachialis muscle and inject 5–7 ml of solution. The usual reason to block the musculocutaneous nerve is to improve sensory block in the territory of its cutaneous distribution – the lateral cutaneous nerve of forearm and this can be done very easily at the elbow instead (pp. 122–123).

The intercostobrachial nerve is not part of the brachial plexus and may need to be blocked separately in the axilla to provide analgesia to the upper, inner aspect of the arm. From the same needle insertion point as for the axillary approach to the brachial plexus, withdraw the needle to the subcutaneous tissues, angle medially and inject 3–5 ml of solution.

Agent	Concn	Volume	Onset	Duration
Bupiv	0.5%	30 ml	40 min	12 h
Prilo	2%	40 ml	20 min	6 h

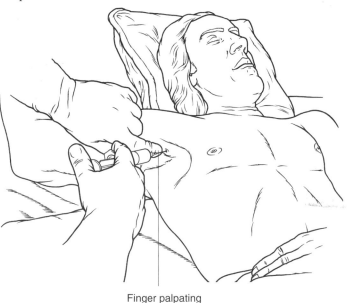

Fig. 3.32.1
Axillary block

Finger palpating
arterial pulse

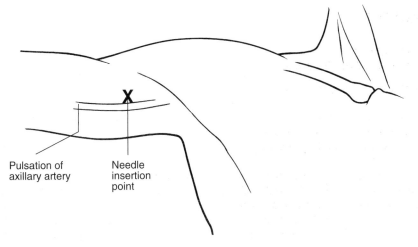

Pulsation of axillary artery

Needle insertion point

Fig. 3.32.2
Axillary block, anterior view

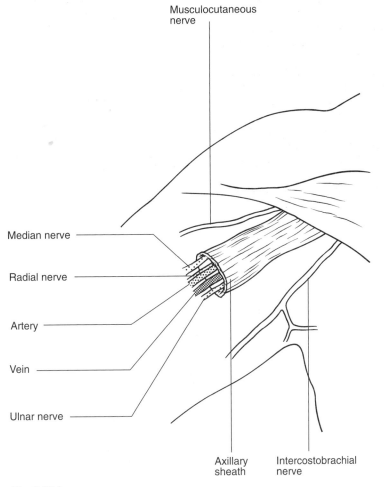

Musculocutaneous nerve

Median nerve

Radial nerve

Artery

Vein

Ulnar nerve

Axillary sheath

Intercostobrachial nerve

Fig. 3.32.3
Axillary block completion, position of musculocutaneous nerve and intercostobrachial nerve

Suprascapular nerve block

Posterior approach

Landmarks
Spine of scapula

The posterior approach is only suitable for conscious patients because the patient must be sat up. Palpate the spine of the scapula and identify the midpoint – the suprascapular notch is approximately 1 cm above it. Insert a 22 G short bevel needle at right angles to the skin to a depth of 2–3 cm at which point bony contact will usually occur (Fig. 3.33.1). Carefully move the needle to locate the edges of the suprascapular notch at which point it will produce paraesthesia in the shoulder if the nerve is contacted (or a peripheral nerve stimulator can be used to locate it). It is important not to insert the needle into the notch to avoid nerve damage and the needle must not be angled superiorly in case it passes anterior to the scapula (Figs 3.33.2, 3.33.3).

Agent	Concn	Volume	Onset	Duration
Bupiv	0.5%	5–7 ml	15 min	6–12 h
Bupiv	0.75%	5–7 ml	10 min	≤24 h

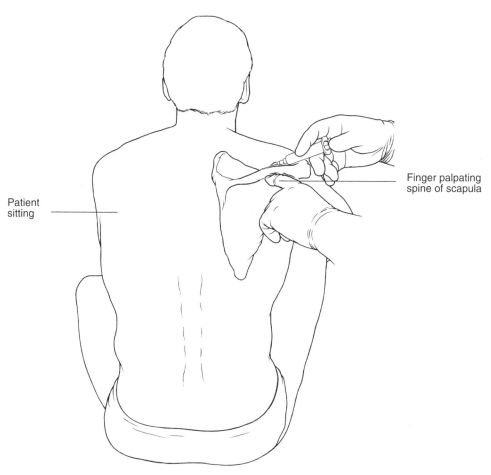

Finger palpating
spine of scapula

Patient
sitting

Fig. 3.33.1
Suprascapular nerve block, posterior approach

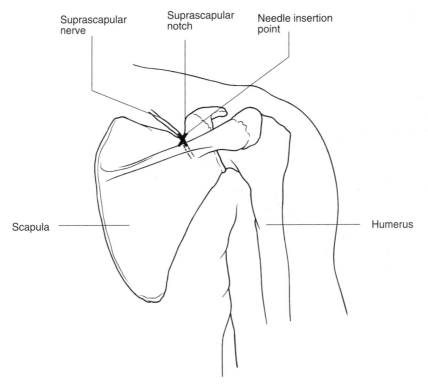

Fig. 3.33.2
Suprascapular nerve block, posterior view

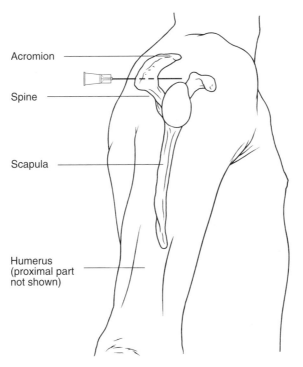

Fig. 3.33.3
Suprascapular nerve block, lateral view

Superior approach

Landmarks
   The acromioclavicular joint

Palpate the medial border of the acromio-clavicular joint. Identification will be made easier if a palpating finger is used to run along the posterior border of the clavicle until no more lateral progress can be made (Figure 3.34.1). At this point a natural groove may be palpated. Insert a 7 cm insulated 22 G short bevel needle aiming for the contralateral nipple. Keep strictly to the saggittal plane and at a depth of 3 cm connect a nerve stimulator and advance the needle tip until pulse synchronous contraction of supraspinatus occurs (Fig. 3.34.1). This will be shown as the initiation of abduction. A common error is too deep placement of the needle (when bone will be felt as the needle

impinges on the medial border of the suprascapular notch). If placement is correct, 5–6 ml of solution is adequate, fade being instant if the needle tip approximates to the nerve. Insulated needles reduce the confusion of unwanted direct stimulation of trapezius which may otherwise be seen (Fig. 3.34.3). For the anterior approach to the suprascapular nerve, see Wasseff (1992).

Agent	Concn	Volume	Onset	Duration
Bupiv	0.5%	5–7 ml	15 min	6–12 h
Bupiv	0.75%	5–7 ml	10 min	≤24 h

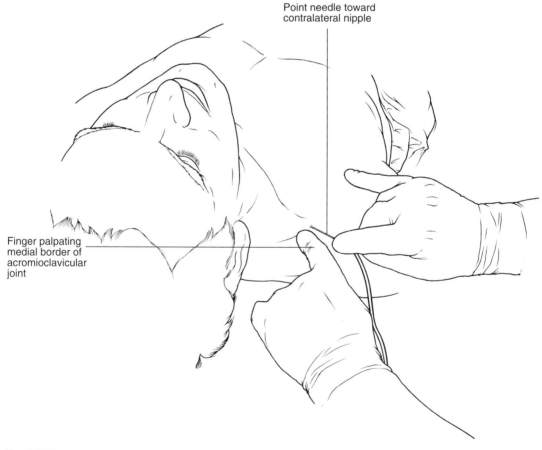

Point needle toward contralateral nipple

Finger palpating medial border of acromioclavicular joint

Fig. 3.34.1
Suprascapular nerve block, superior approach

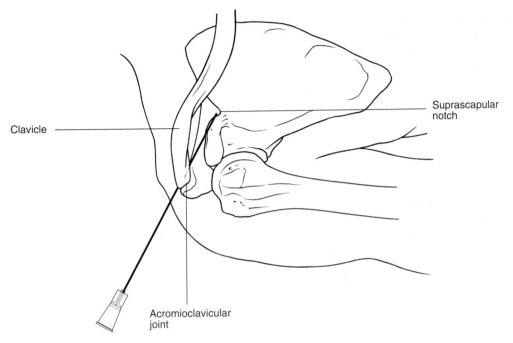

Clavicle

Suprascapular notch

Acromioclavicular joint

Fig. 3.34.2
Suprascapular nerve block, anterior view (rib cage not shown)

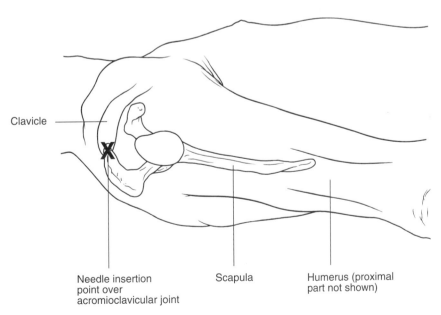

Clavicle

Needle insertion point over acromioclavicular joint

Scapula

Humerus (proximal part not shown)

Fig. 3.34.3
Suprascapular nerve block, lateral view

Nerve blockade at the elbow

The ulnar, median and radial nerves may be approached singly or in combination at the elbow to provide sensory loss to the hand and motor loss to the forearm muscles and the intrinsic muscles of the hand. If sensory loss to the forearm is required, then the lateral, medial and posterior cutaneous nerves of the forearm must be blocked separately at the elbow.

Ulnar nerve block

Landmarks
   Medial epicondyle of humerus
   Ulnar sulcus

Abduct the arm to 90°at the shoulder, supinate the forearm and flex the elbow to 90° (Fig. 3.35.1). Palpate the medial epicondyle of the humerus. It is often possible to 'roll' the nerve beneath the palpating finger just proximal to the epicondyle before the nerve enters the sulcus behind the condyle. Insert a 22 G short bevel needle 1–2 cm proximal to the epicondyle in the horizontal plane (Figs 3.35.2, 3.35.3) and gently advance until paraesthesiae are elicited or until the needle strikes bone in which case withdraw slightly and reposition. The nerve is superficial and the needle rarely needs to be inserted more than 0.5–1.0 cm. Inject 3–4 ml of solution slowly. The injection should be of low resistance and cause no pain or paraesthesiae. Resistance to injection or pain indicates intraneural injection and the injection should be stopped immediately and the needle repositioned. If the nerve is difficult to locate, a peripheral nerve stimulator may be used to confirm its position when pulse synchronous flexion of fingers and wrist will be seen.

To avoid the possibility of nerve damage, do not look for the nerve within the ulnar nerve sulcus of the medial epicondyle. At this point, the nerve is tightly restricted by the medial ligament of the elbow and thus cannot move away from the advancing needle tip. It may also be exposed to high pressure ischaemic damage if a large volume of solution is injected into this small channel.

Agent	Concn	Volume	Onset	Duration
Bupiv	0.5%	4 ml	10 min	12 h
Prilo	1%	4 ml	10 min	4 h

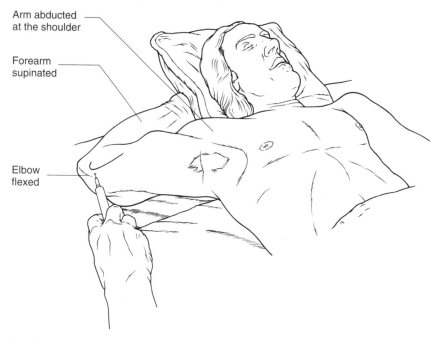

Arm abducted at the shoulder

Forearm supinated

Elbow flexed

Fig. 3.35.1
Ulnar nerve block

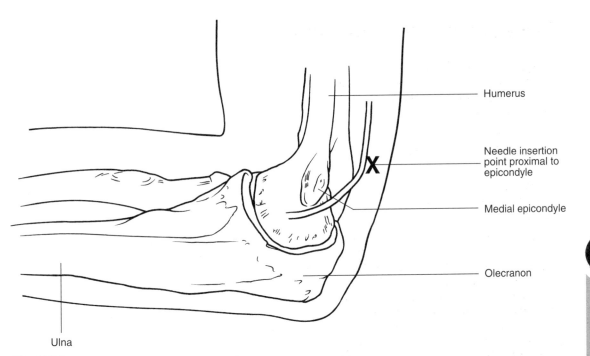

Humerus

Needle insertion point proximal to epicondyle

Medial epicondyle

Olecranon

Ulna

Fig. 3.35.2
Ulnar nerve block, medial view

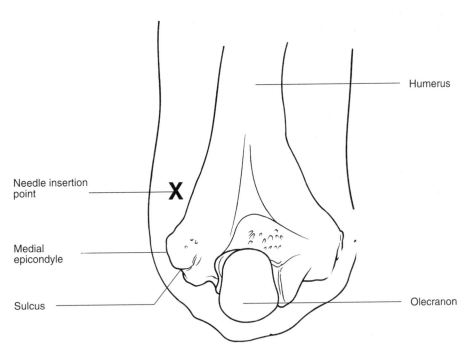

Humerus

Needle insertion point

Medial epicondyle

Sulcus

Olecranon

Fig. 3.35.3
Ulnar nerve block, posterior view

Technique   **119**

Median nerve block

Landmarks
  Antecubital fossa
  Brachial artery pulse
  Medial border of biceps tendon
  Humoral head of pronator teres

Abduct the arm at an angle of 45° and hold it in extension with the patient positioned supine (Fig. 3.36.1). Between the biceps tendon and the head of pronator teres is an intermuscular groove in which the brachial artery is palpable just proximal to the flexor crease of the antecubital fossa (Fig. 3.36.2). Having identified the brachial artery, insert a 22 G short bevel needle at an angle of 45° to the skin just medial to the brachial artery and 1–2 cm proximal to the flexor skin crease of the antecubital fossa (Fig. 3.36.2). There may be a 'pop' or loss of resistance as the needle penetrates the bicipital aponeurosis beneath which the nerve lies. After the onset of paraesthesiae inject 4–5 ml of solution slowly. A peripheral nerve stimulator may be used to locate the nerve when pulse synchronous flexion of fingers and wrist will be seen.

Agent	Concn	Volume	Onset	Duration
Bupiv	0.5%	5 ml	10 min	12 h
Prilo	1%	5 ml	10 min	4 h

Medial cutaneous nerve of forearm block

Landmarks
  See median nerve block

The medial cutaneous nerve of the forearm is usually blocked in conjunction with the median nerve and requires the same landmarks. On completion of the median nerve block, withdraw the needle to the subcutaneous tissue and then advance proximally along the intermuscular groove whilst injecting a 'sausage' of up to 7 ml of solution (Fig. 3.36.3).

Agent	Concn	Volume	Onset	Duration
Bupiv	0.25%	5–7 ml	15 min	6 h

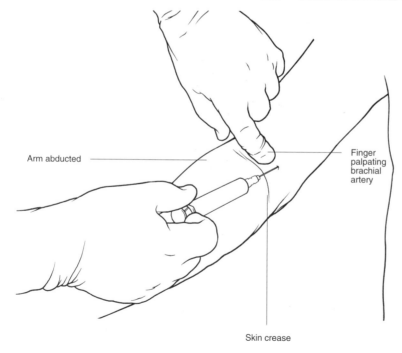

Arm abducted

Finger palpating brachial artery

Skin crease

Fig. 3.36.1
Median nerve block

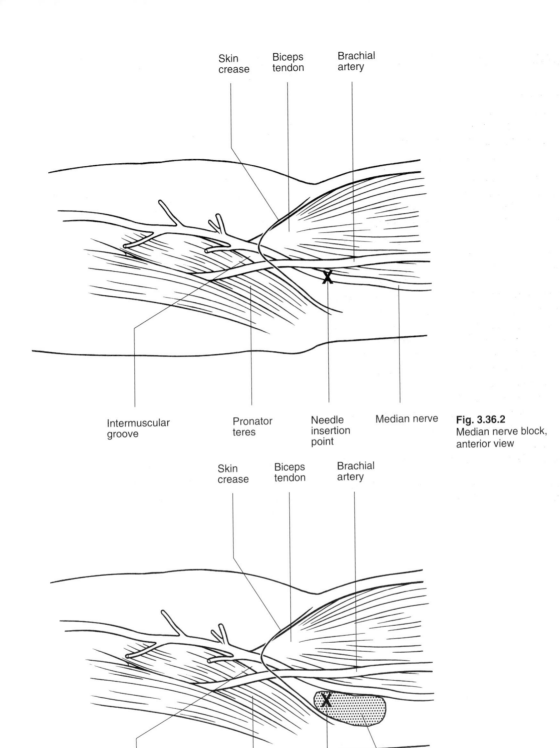

Skin crease | Biceps tendon | Brachial artery

Intermuscular groove | Pronator teres | Needle insertion point | Median nerve

Fig. 3.36.2
Median nerve block, anterior view

Skin crease | Biceps tendon | Brachial artery

Intermuscular groove | Pronator teres | Needle insertion point | Subcutaneous sausage of solution

Fig. 3.36.3
Medial cutaneous nerve of forearm, anterior view

Radial nerve block

Landmarks
- Antecubital fossa
- Lateral epicondyle of humerus
- Lateral border of biceps tendon
- Medial border of brachioradialis muscle

Hold the arm with the elbow extended and identify the intermuscular groove between the biceps and brachioradialis just proximal to the flexor skin crease of the antecubital fossa (Fig. 3.37.1). The nerve runs deep to the brachioradialis muscle at this point and can be difficult to locate, especially if relying on paraesthesiae. Use of a peripheral nerve stimulator will aid location (motor response will be extension of fingers and wrist) and improve success when attempting this technique. Identify the lateral epicondyle and place a finger on this landmark to act as a guide for the direction of needle insertion. Insert a 3.5 cm 22 G short bevel needle into the intermuscular groove approximately 2 cm proximal to the flexor skin crease of the antecubital fossa and aim towards the lateral epicondyle (Fig. 3.37.2). Paraesthesiae (or pulse synchronous movement in the distribution of the nerve) may occur before the needle strikes bone in which case 5–7 ml of solution should be injected. Otherwise the needle must be redirected more medially until the nerve is found.

Agent	Concn	Volume	Onset	Duration
Bupiv	0.5%	7 ml	15 min	12 h
Prilo	1%	10 ml	15 min	4 h

Lateral cutaneous nerve of forearm block

Landmarks
- See radial nerve block

The lateral cutaneous nerve of forearm is usually blocked in conjunction with the radial nerve and the same landmarks are required. After completion of the radial nerve block, withdraw the needle so that it is just deep to the deep fascia and lateral to the biceps tendon in the intermuscular groove (Fig. 3.37.3). Re-angle the needle to lie parallel with the tendon and inject 5–7 ml of solution.

Agent	Concn	Volume	Onset	Duration
Bupiv	0.25%	5–7 ml	15 min	12 h
Prilo	1%	5–7 ml	15 min	4 h

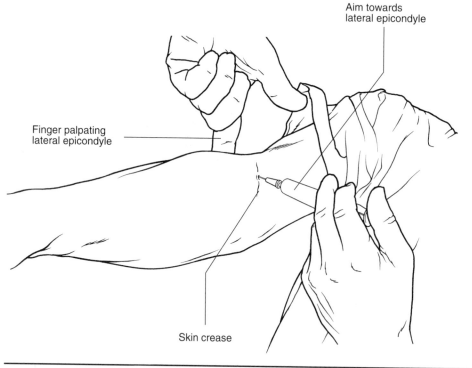

Aim towards lateral epicondyle

Finger palpating lateral epicondyle

Skin crease

Fig. 3.37.1
Radial nerve block

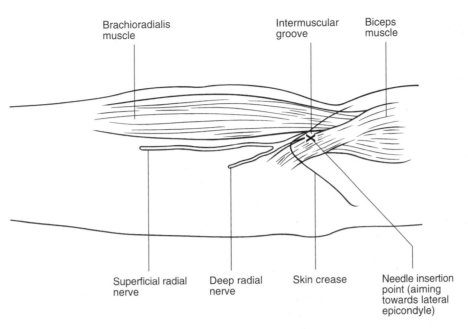

Fig. 3.37.2
Radial nerve block, anterior view

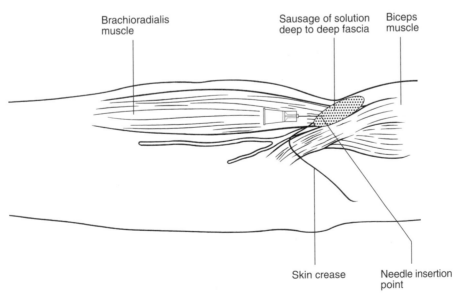

Fig. 3.37.3
Lateral cutaneous nerve of forearm block, anterior view

Posterior cutaneous nerve of forearm block

Landmarks
> Lateral epicondyle of humerus
> Olecranon process

Flex the arm across the chest of the patient and, from a point directly over the lateral epicondyle, inject a subcutaneous 'sausage' of solution medially until the olecranon process is reached (Figs 3.38.1, 3.38.2, 3.38.3).

Agent	Concn	Volume	Onset	Duration
Bupiv	0.25%	5 ml	10 min	12 h
Prilo	1%	5 ml	10 min	4 h

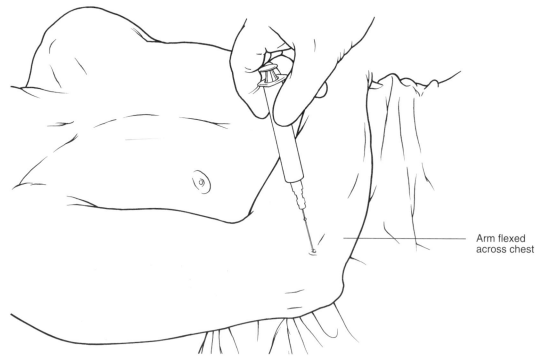

Arm flexed
across chest

Fig. 3.38.1
Posterior cutaneous nerve of forearm block

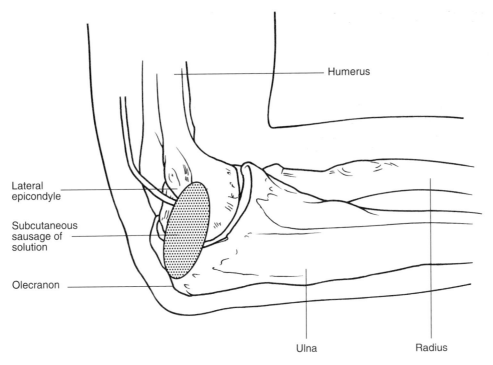

Fig. 3.38.2
Posterior cutaneous nerve of forearm block, lateral view

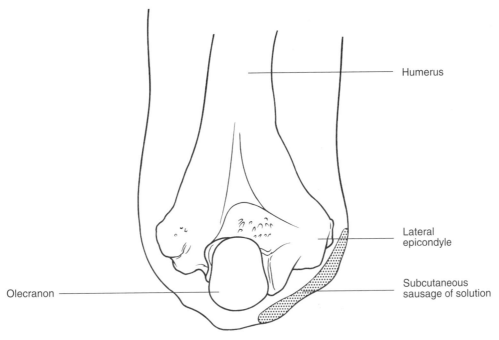

Fig. 3.38.3
Posterior cutaneous nerve of forearm block, posterior view

Nerve blockade at the wrist

Nerve blockade at the wrist will produce sensory loss of the hand and motor loss of the intrinsic muscles of the hand (but not of the extensors and flexors of the hand and wrist).

Ulnar nerve block

There are two methods of approaching the nerve, ventral and medial. The medial approach is preferable because ulnar artery damage is less likely as it lies lateral to the nerve. Additionally, both the dorsal and palmar cutaneous branches may be blocked from the same needle insertion point.

Ventral approach

Landmarks
   Flexor carpi ulnaris tendon
   Ulnar artery pulse
   Pisiform bone

Place the arm supine and identify the flexor carpi ulnaris tendon approximately 1 cm proximal to its insertion into the pisiform at the skin crease of the wrist. It is usually possible to palpate the ulnar artery at this point and the ulnar nerve lies medial to the artery and deep to the radial border of the tendon. Advance a 25 G needle perpendicular to the skin between the flexor carpi ulnaris tendon and the ulnar artery pulsation (Fig. 3.39.1) until paraesthesiae are elicited approximately 1 cm deep to the skin.

Slowly inject 3–4 ml of solution and then withdraw the needle to the subcutaneous tissue where a further 2–3 ml should be injected to block the palmar cutaneous branch (Figs 3.39.2, 3.39.3).

Agent	Concn	Volume	Onset	Duration
Bupiv	0.25%	7 ml	10 min	6–12 h
Prilo	1%	7 ml	10 min	4 h

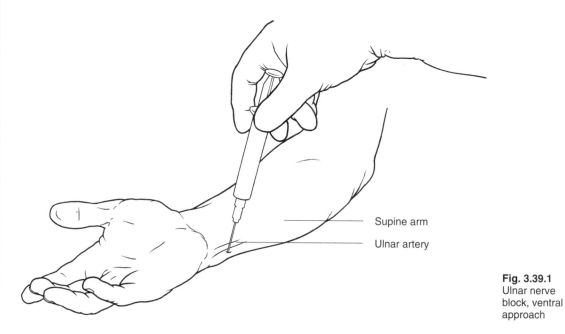

Supine arm

Ulnar artery

Fig. 3.39.1
Ulnar nerve block, ventral approach

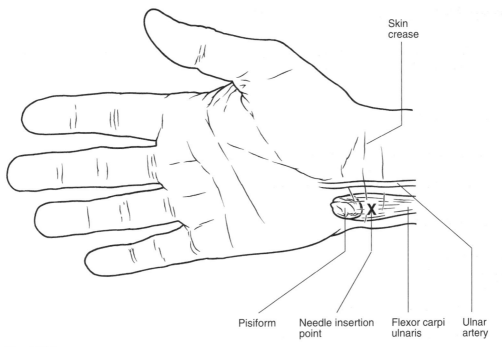

Skin
crease

X

Pisiform

Needle insertion
point

Flexor carpi
ulnaris

Ulnar
artery

Fig. 3.39.2
Ulnar nerve block, palmar view

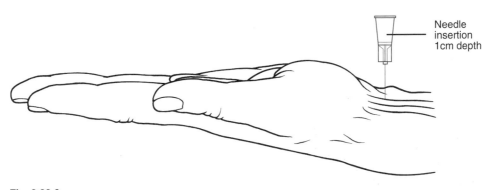

Needle
insertion
1cm depth

Fig. 3.39.3
Ulnar nerve block, medial view

Medial approach

Landmarks
Flexor carpi ulnaris tendon
Ulnar artery pulse
Pisiform bone

With the wrist supine and abducted from the body, insert a 25 G needle at 90° to the skin immediately deep to the flexor carpi ulnaris tendon, about 1 cm proximal to the pisiform bone (Fig. 3.40.1). At a depth of 1–1.5 cm, slowly inject 3–4 ml of solution and withdraw the needle to the subcutaneous tissue where it should then be redirected both dorsally to block the dorsal branch with 2 ml of solution and ventrally to block the palmar branch with 2 ml of solution (Figs 3.40.2, 3.40.3).

Agent	Concn	Volume	Onset	Duration
Bupiv	0.25%	8 ml	20 min	6–12 h
Prilo	1%	8 ml	10 min	4 h
Lido	1%	8 ml	5 min	3 h

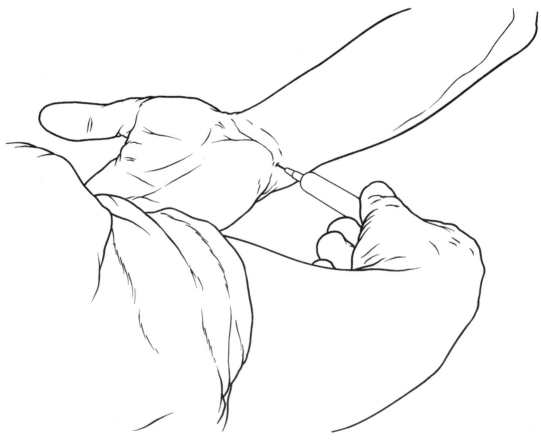

Fig. 3.40.1
Ulnar nerve block, medial approach

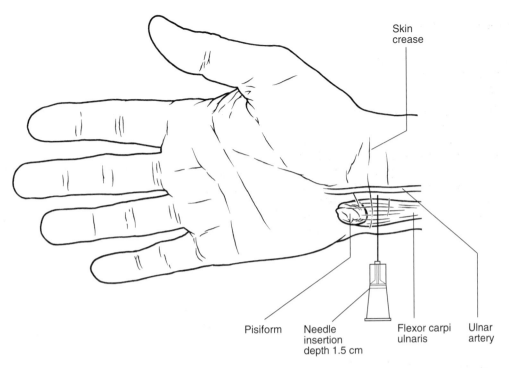

Fig. 3.40.2
Ulnar nerve block, ventral or palmar view

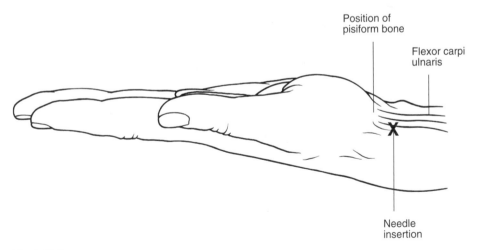

Fig. 3.40.3
Ulnar nerve block, medial view

Median nerve block

Landmarks
  Flexor carpi radialis tendon
  Palmaris longus tendon (if present)

Position the wrist supine and slightly abducted. The palmaris tendon can be highlighted by asking the patient to flex the wrist against resistance and, if it is present, insert a 25 G needle just lateral to the tendon (Fig. 3.41.1). In the absence of palmaris longus, insert the needle 1 cm medial to the ulnar border of flexor carpi radialis tendon. At a depth of up to 1 cm, increased resistance indicates that the flexor retinaculum has been reached and the needle should be slowly advanced a further 2–3 mm. The nerve lies immediately deep to the retinaculum and as soon as paraesthesiae are elicited, immobilise the needle and carefully inject 3–4 ml of solution. Resistance to injection or pain may indicate intraneural injection in which case stop and reposition the needle. On completion of the median nerve block, withdraw the needle to the subcutaneous tissue and inject a further 2 ml of solution to block the palmar cutaneous branch (Figs 3.41.2, 3.41.3).

Note. Do not use this approach in the presence of carpal tunnel syndrome due to the tight restriction of the nerve beneath the retinaculum.

Agent	Concn	Volume	Onset	Duration
Bupiv	0.25%	6 ml	20 min	6 h
Prilo	1%	6 ml	10 min	4 h
Lido	1%	6 ml	5 min	2 h

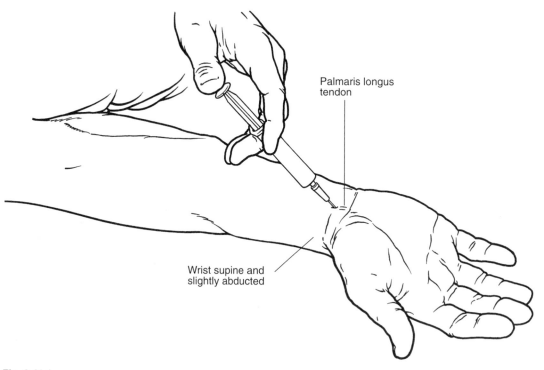

Palmaris longus tendon

Wrist supine and slightly abducted

Fig. 3.41.1
Median nerve block

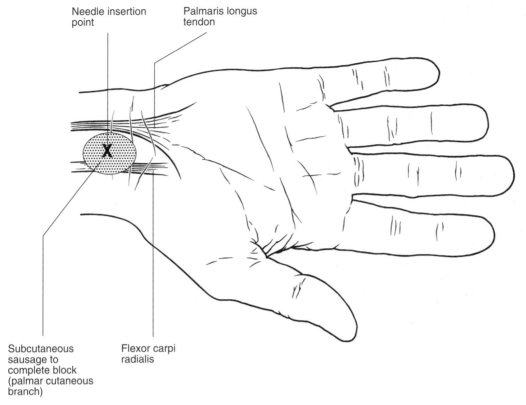

Needle insertion point

Palmaris longus tendon

Subcutaneous sausage to complete block (palmar cutaneous branch)

Flexor carpi radialis

Fig. 3.41.2
Median nerve block, ventral or palmar view

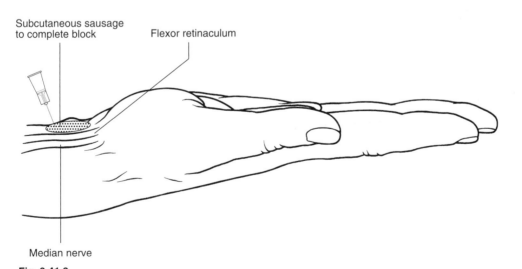

Subcutaneous sausage to complete block

Flexor retinaculum

Median nerve

Fig. 3.41.3
Median nerve block, lateral view

Radial nerve block

Landmarks
Styloid process of ulna
Styloid process of radius
Tendon of extensor pollicis brevis
Tendon of extensor pollicis longus

Position the arm prone and abducted from the body. If the thumb is extended against resistance, the tendons will be thrown into relief and the 'anatomical snuff box' can be identified, overlying the styloid process of the radius. At this level, the radial nerve is subcutaneous and has already divided into its terminal branches to the thumb and radial aspect of the dorsum of the hand. Insert a 22 G 3.5 cm needle close to the tendon of extensor pollicis longus over the styloid process of the radius and direct it subcutaneously across the dorsum of the wrist towards the ulnar border of the wrist along a line joining both styloid processes (Fig. 3.42.1). Inject a 5–7 ml 'sausage' of solution as the needle is advanced (Fig. 3.42.2). Withdraw the needle to the insertion point and redirect it across the tendon of flexor pollicis brevis and inject a further 2–3 ml of solution subcutaneously. This technique may more properly be considered a field block rather than a discrete nerve block (Figs 3.42.3, 3.42.4).

Agent	Concn	Volume	Onset	Duration
Bupiv	0.5%	10 ml	20 min	12 h
Bupiv	0.25%	10 ml	20 min	6 h
Prilo	1%	10 ml	15 min	4 h
Lido	1%	10 ml	5 min	2 h

Fig. 3.42.1
Radial nerve block

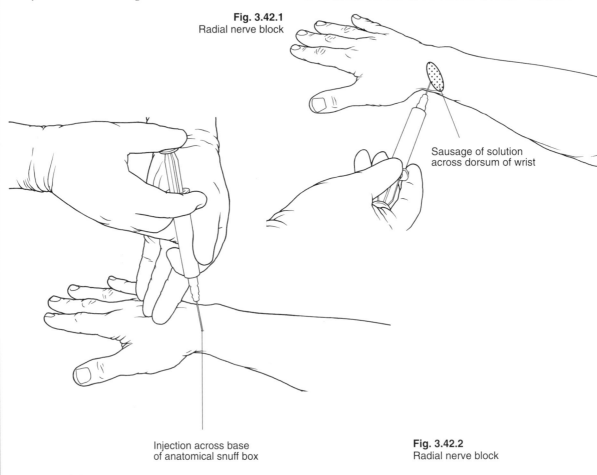

Sausage of solution
across dorsum of wrist

Injection across base
of anatomical snuff box

Fig. 3.42.2
Radial nerve block

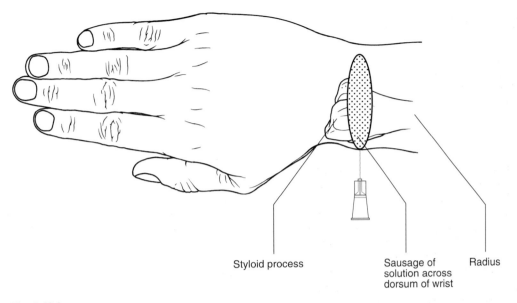

Styloid process   Sausage of   Radius
solution across
dorsum of wrist

Fig. 3.42.3
Radial nerve block, dorsal view

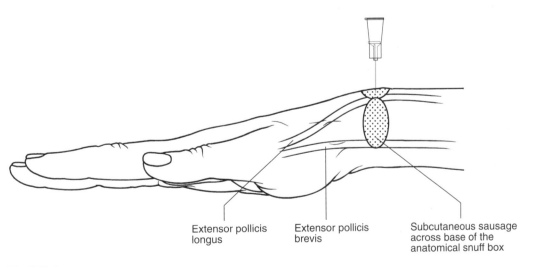

Extensor pollicis   Extensor pollicis   Subcutaneous sausage
longus   brevis   across base of the
anatomical snuff box

Fig. 3.42.4
Radial nerve block, medial view

Digital nerve block

There are three approaches to the digital nerves of the hand: metacarpal, classical and web space. The metacarpal approach is perhaps more painful for the patient and should be reserved for those occasions when anaesthesia of the intrinsic muscles and other deep structures of the hand is required. When anaesthesia of the fingers alone is required, the classical dorsal approach to the digital nerves or the web space approach are equally satisfactory, although the latter is more comfortable for the conscious patient.

Metacarpal block

Landmarks
   Intermetacarpal spaces

Place the hand prone and identify the intermetacarpal spaces corresponding to the fingers to be blocked at their midpoints. Insert a 25 G needle perpendicular to the skin and direct it vertically towards the palmar surface of the hand (Fig. 3.43.1). Place a finger on the palm beneath the space to detect the needle as it approaches the palmar aponeurosis which it should not pierce because the digital nerves lie deep to the aponeurosis. Inject 2 ml of solution at the aponeurosis, a further 2 ml as the needle is withdrawn and then a final 2 ml at the level of the dorsal border of the metacarpal (Figs 3.43.2, 3.43.3).

Agent	Concn	Volume	Onset	Duration
Bupiv	0.5%	6 ml	20 min	12 h
Prilo	1%	6 ml	20 min	4 h

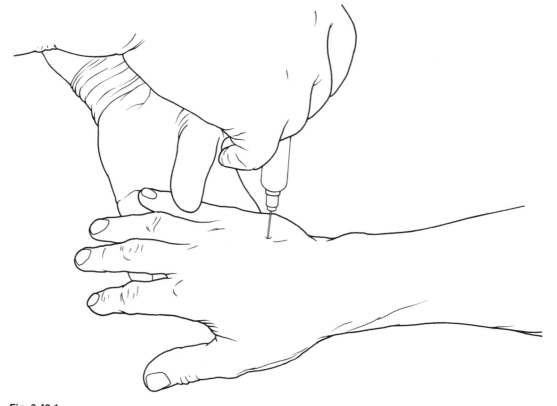

Fig. 3.43.1
Digital nerve block, metacarpal approach

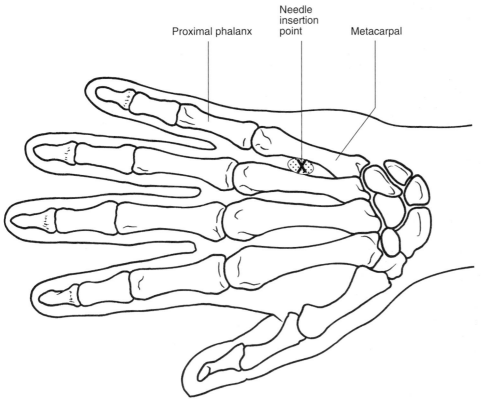

Proximal phalanx   Needle insertion point   Metacarpal

Fig. 3.43.2
Metacarpal block, dorsal view

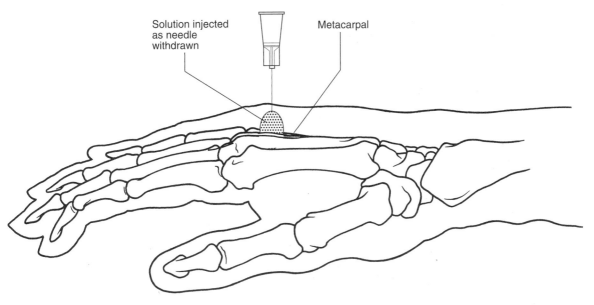

Solution injected as needle withdrawn   Metacarpal

Fig. 3.43.3
Metatarsal block, medial view

Digital nerve block

Landmarks
  Metacarpo-phalangeal joints
  Web spaces

With the hand prone, identify the appropriate metacarpo-phalangeal joints and insert a 25 G needle perpendicular to the skin, just distal to the joint. Place a finger on the palmar surface to detect the needle as it advances towards the palmar border of the phalanx (Fig. 3.44.1). With the needle at its deepest position slowly inject 3 ml of solution as the needle is withdrawn (Figs 3.44.2, 3.44.3).

Agent	Concn	Volume	Onset	Duration
Bupiv	0.5%	3 ml	20 min	12 h

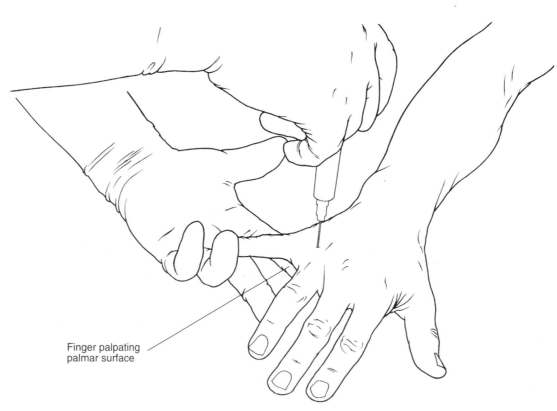

Finger palpating palmar surface

Fig. 3.44.1
Digital nerve block, classical approach

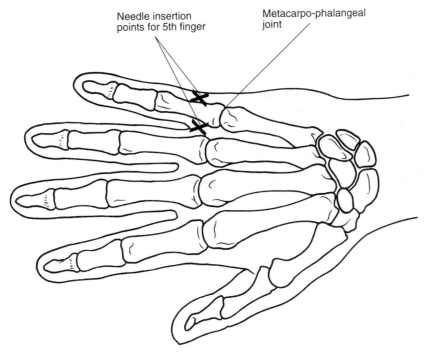

Needle insertion
points for 5th finger

Metacarpo-phalangeal
joint

Fig. 3.44.2
Digital nerve block, dorsal view

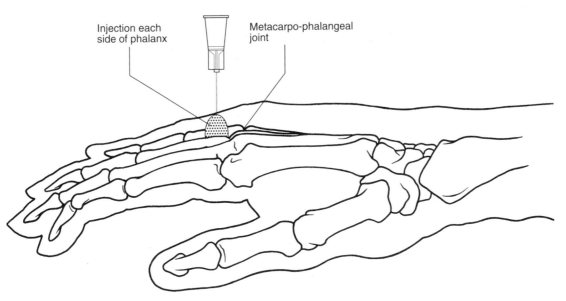

Injection each
side of phalanx

Metacarpo-phalangeal
joint

Fig. 3.44.3
Digital nerve block, medial view

Web space block

Landmarks
  Web spaces

Approach the digital nerves in the horizontal plane by separating the fingers that delimit the space and insert a 25 G needle into the web space to a depth of 2 cm until the needle tip is level with the metacarpo-phalangeal joint (Figs 3.54.1, 3.54.2). After negative aspiration, inject 5 ml of solution. There should be no resistance to injection but the web space will distend slightly. Gently massage the space to disperse the solution around the dorsal and ventral nerves after removing the needle. To avoid causing ischaemia to the digits, do not use local anaesthetic solutions which contain vasoconstrictors. Hydraulic pressure ischaemia due to large volume injection should be avoided by limiting the volume to 5 ml per space or less.

Agent	Concn	Volume	Onset	Duration
Bupiv	0.5%	5 ml	20 min	12 h

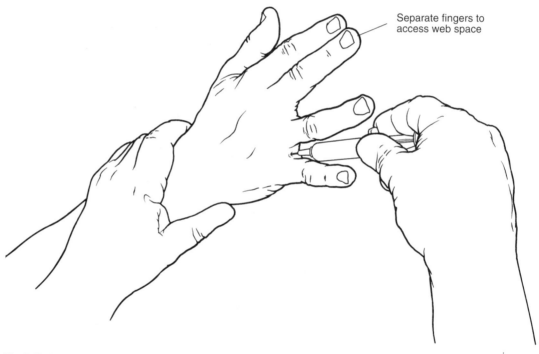

Separate fingers to access web space

Fig. 3.45.1
Web space block

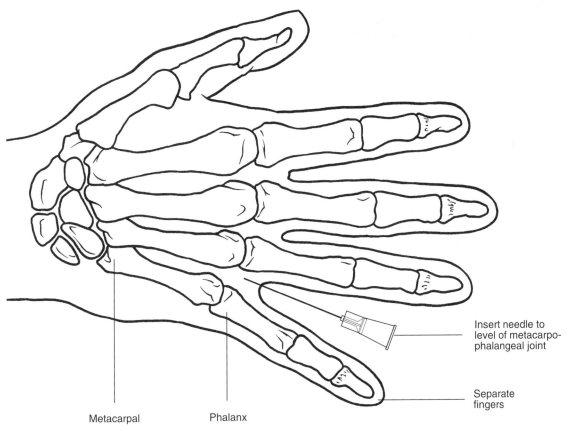

Insert needle to
level of metacarpo-
phalangeal joint

Separate
fingers

Metacarpal   Phalanx

Fig. 3.45.2
Web space block, dorsal view

Superficial cervical plexus block

Landmarks
  Posterior border of sternomastoid
  Cricoid cartilage

Position the patient supine with the head turned slightly to the opposite side, as in Figure 3.46.1. A line drawn laterally from the cricoid cartilage usually crosses the posterior border of the sternomastoid muscle at the point at which the nerves of the plexus emerge (Fig. 3.46.2). If the posterior border is difficult to identify, ask the patient to raise their head from the pillow slightly with it still turned away from the side to be blocked. Insert a 22 G short bevel needle immediately behind the muscle at right angles

to the skin until it 'pops' through the cervical fascia (Fig. 3.46.3). If the needle is in the correct tissue plane, an injection of 10 ml of local anaesthetic will be seen to flow up and down the posterior border of the muscle.

Agent	Concn	Volume	Onset	Duration
Bupiv	0.5%	10 ml	20 min	12 h
Prilo	1%	10 ml	10 min	4 h

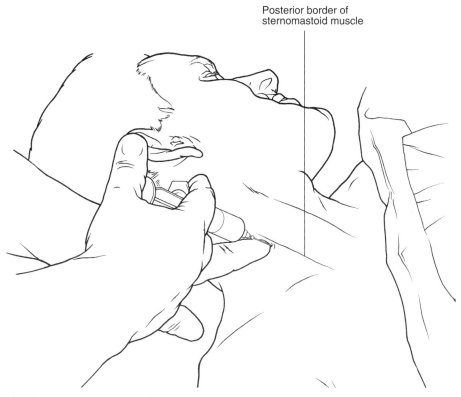

Posterior border of
sternomastoid muscle

Fig. 3.46.1
Superficial cervical plexus block

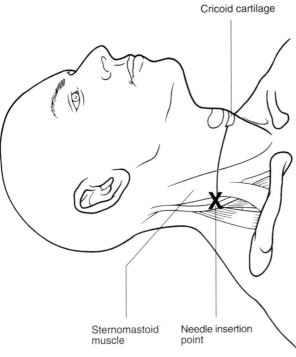

Cricoid cartilage

X

Sternomastoid
muscle

Needle insertion
point

Fig. 3.46.2
Superficial cervical plexus block, lateral view

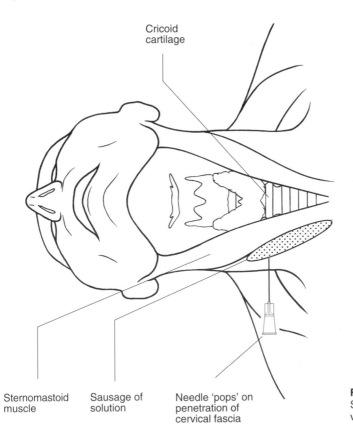

Cricoid
cartilage

Sternomastoid
muscle

Sausage of
solution

Needle 'pops' on
penetration of
cervical fascia

Fig. 3.46.3
Superficial cervical plexus block, anterior
view

Technique   141

Greater and lesser occipital nerve block

The lesser occipital nerve and the greater auricular nerve can be blocked either as part of a cervical plexus block or they can be blocked separately for operations on the scalp and ear.

Landmarks
Greater occipital protuberance
Mastoid process
Posterior occipital artery

Position the patient's head so that the occipital protuberance and the mastoid process can be palpated and a line between them defined. Insert a 25 G needle subcutaneously 2 cm lateral to the occipital protuberance to travel along the line between the bony landmarks (the pulsation of the artery, which accompanies the greater occipital nerve may be palpable at this point). Inject 4–5 ml of solution at this point and then redirect the needle along the line and inject a further 3–4 ml subcutaneously towards the mastoid process to block the lesser occipital nerve (Figs 3.47.1, 3.47.2).

Agent	Concn	Volume	Onset	Duration
Bupiv	0.25%	7–9 ml	10 min	6 h
Prilo	1%	7–9 ml	6 min	4 h

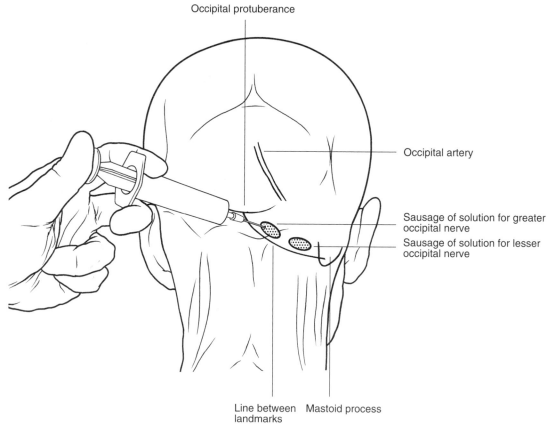

Occipital protuberance

Occipital artery

Sausage of solution for greater occipital nerve

Sausage of solution for lesser occipital nerve

Line between landmarks   Mastoid process

Fig. 3.47.1
Greater and lesser occipital nerve block

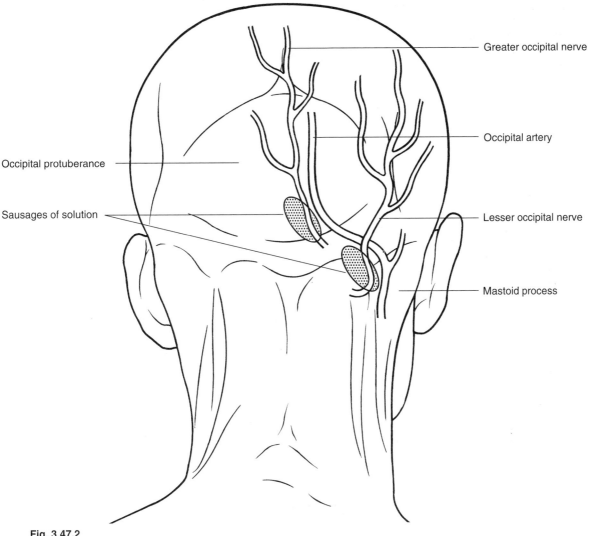

Occipital protuberance

Sausages of solution

Greater occipital nerve

Occipital artery

Lesser occipital nerve

Mastoid process

Fig. 3.47.2
Greater and lesser occipital nerve block, posterior view

Greater auricular nerve block

Landmarks
Mastoid process

Turn the head away from the side to be blocked and using a 25 G needle, infiltrate 7–10 ml of solution along the posterior aspect of the mastoid process (Fig. 3.48.1).

Agent	Concn	Volume	Onset	Duration
Bupiv + adren	0.25%	7–10 ml	10 min	6–8 h

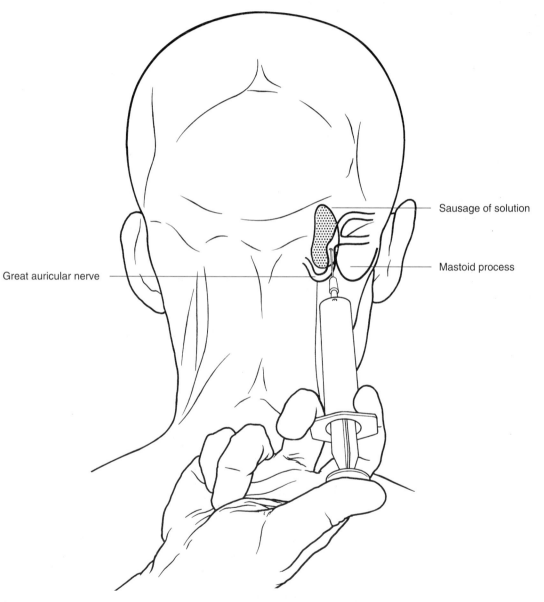

Sausage of solution

Mastoid process

Great auricular nerve

Fig. 3.48.1
Great auricular nerve block

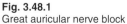

Auriculotemporal nerve block

Landmarks
  Superficial temporal artery
  Temporomandibular joint
  Tragus of ear

The auriculotemporal nerve accompanies the artery which can be palpated superior to the temporomandibular joint. Insert a 25 G needle at right angles to the skin between the pulsation of the artery and the tragus and after careful negative aspiration, inject 4–6 ml of solution (Figs 3.49.1, 3.49.2).

Agent	Concn	Volume	Onset	Duration
Prilo	1%	4–6 ml	5–6 min	3–4 h
Bupiv	0.25%	4–6 ml	10 min	4–6 h

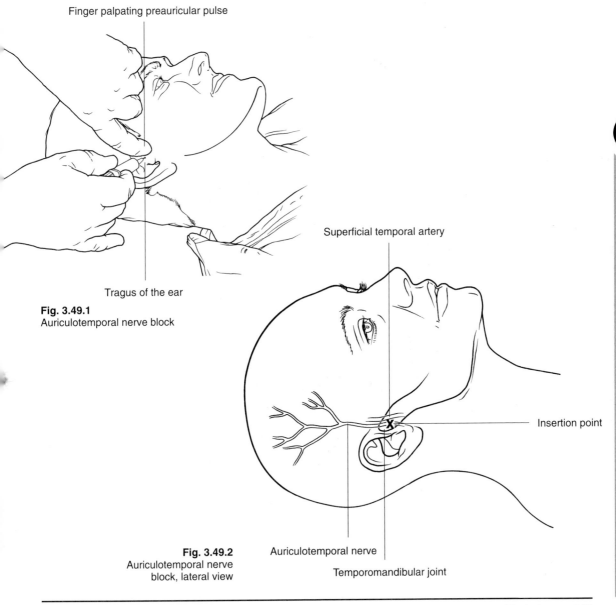

Finger palpating preauricular pulse

Tragus of the ear

Fig. 3.49.1
Auriculotemporal nerve block

Superficial temporal artery

Insertion point

Fig. 3.49.2
Auriculotemporal nerve block, lateral view

Auriculotemporal nerve

Temporomandibular joint

Zygomaticofacial and zygomaticotemporal nerve blocks

These nerves have limited territories and are usually blocked in combination.

Landmarks
   Zygomaticofacial foramen
   Lateral border of orbit

The zygomaticofacial foramen can usually be palpated 1 cm or so below the lateral border of the orbit. Use a 25 G needle to make a subcutaneous injection of 2–3 ml of solution around the branches of the nerve as they emerge from the foramen and then redirect the needle subcutaneously upwards and slightly backwards along the lateral border of the orbit and inject a further 2–3 ml to block the zygomaticotemporal nerve (Figs 3.50.1, 3.50.2).

Agent	Concn	Volume	Onset	Duration
Prilo	1%	4–6 ml	5 min	3–4 h
Bupiv	0.25%	4–6 ml	10 min	4–6 h

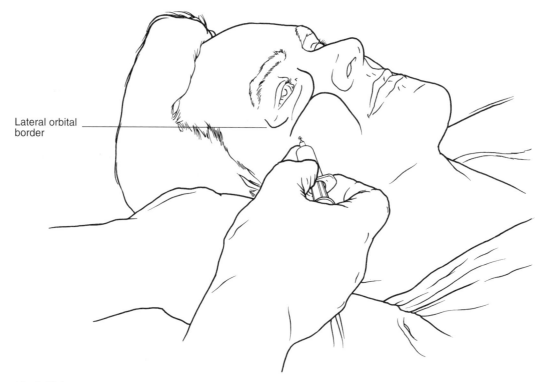

Lateral orbital border

Fig. 3.50.1
Zygomaticofacial and zygomaticotemporal nerve blocks

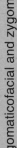

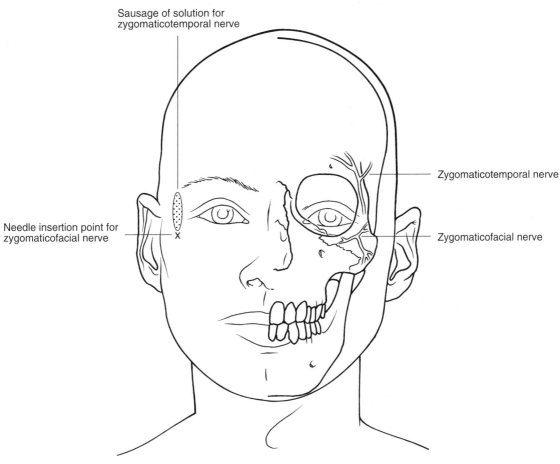

Sausage of solution for
zygomaticotemporal nerve

Zygomaticotemporal nerve

Needle insertion point for
zygomaticofacial nerve

Zygomaticofacial nerve

Fig. 3.50.2
Zygomaticofacial and zygomaticotemporal blocks, anterior view

Blockade for anterior facial nerves

The three foraminae for the mental nerve, infraorbital nerve and supraorbital blocks all lie in the same plane which passes through the pupil when the eye is held in its primary midpoint resting position (Fig. 3.51.2).

Mental nerve block

Landmarks
  Mental foramen

Palpate the mental foramen of the mandible and introduce a 25 G needle subcutaneously towards the foramen (Fig. 3.51.1). It is not necessary to enter the foramen. A single injection of 2–3 ml of solution in proximity to foramen is sufficient (Figure 3.51.2).

Agent	Concn	Volume	Onset	Duration
Bupiv	0.25%	3 ml	10 min	6 h
Prilo	1%	3 ml	6 min	4 h

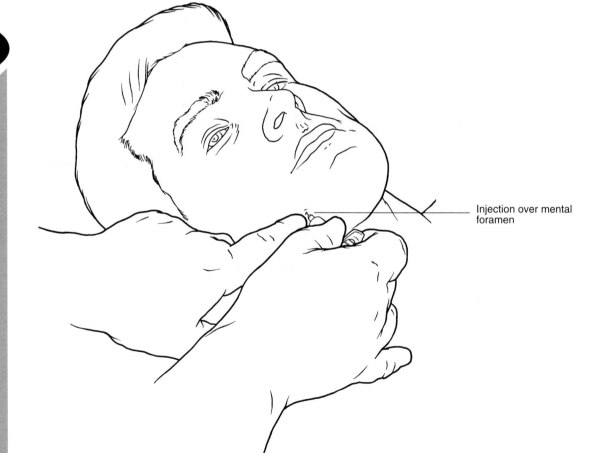

Injection over mental foramen

Fig. 3.51.1
Mental nerve block

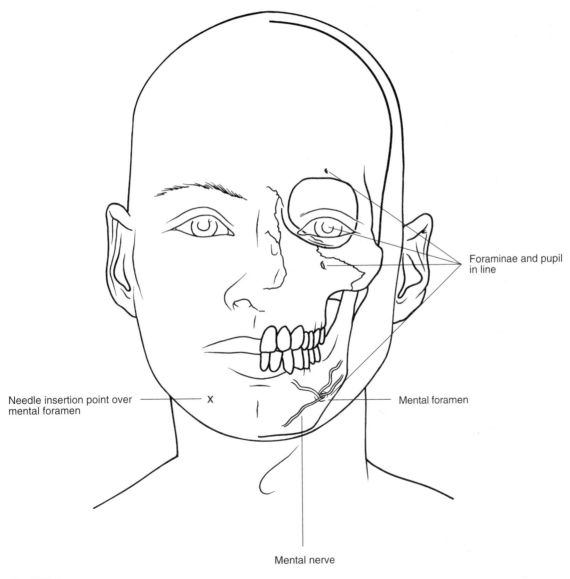

Foraminae and pupil
in line

Needle insertion point over
mental foramen

X

Mental foramen

Mental nerve

Fig. 3.51.2
Mental nerve block, anterior view

Infraorbital nerve block

Landmarks
Infraorbital foramen

Palpate the infraorbital foramen, which lies approximately 1 cm below the midpoint of the lower border of the orbit and 1 cm lateral to the external nares. Insert a 25 G needle subcutaneously towards the foramen and inject 2–3 ml of solution around the outlet of the foramen (Figs 3.52.1, 3.52.2). It is important not to introduce the needle into the nerve canal as the nerve and the floor of the orbit can be damaged.

Agent	Concn	Volume	Onset	Duration
Bupiv	0.25%	3 ml	10 min	6 h
Prilo	1%	3 ml	6 min	4 h

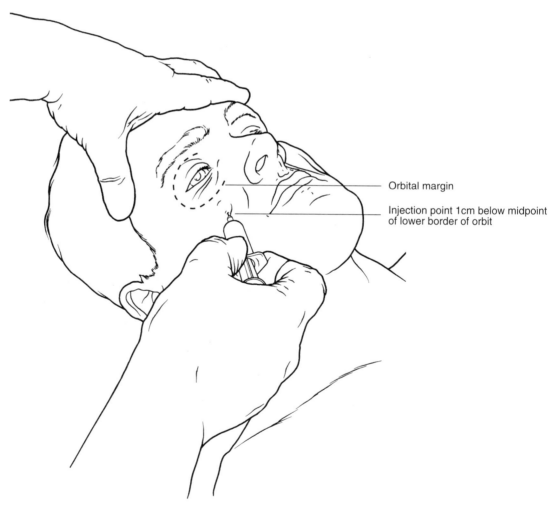

Orbital margin

Injection point 1cm below midpoint of lower border of orbit

Fig. 3.52.1
Infraorbital nerve block

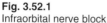
Head and neck
Infraorbital nerve block

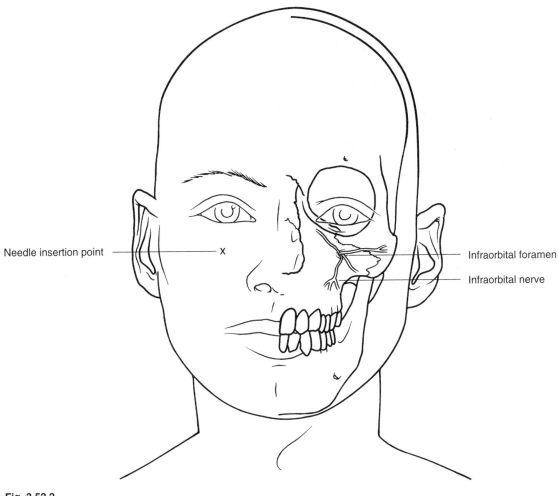

Needle insertion point —————————— X

Infraorbital foramen

Infraorbital nerve

Fig. 3.52.2
Infraorbital nerve block, anterior view

Supraorbital and supratrochlear nerve blocks

These nerves are usually blocked together because of their proximity and overlapping territories.

Landmarks
    Supraorbital notch
    Bridge of nose

Palpate the supraorbital notch, which lies at the approximate mid point of the superior border of the orbit and insert a 25 G needle subcutaneously as in Figure 3.53.1 so that the tip just touches the periosteum of the frontal bone. Withdraw the needle very slightly and slowly inject 3–4 ml of solution. Re-angle medially and inject a further 2–3 ml of solution as a subcutaneous 'sausage' while advancing the needle medially along the orbital border as far as the bridge of the nose (Figs 3.53.1, 3.53.2, 3.53.3).

For bilateral anaesthesia, use a mid-point injection on the bridge of the nose, through a skin weal of local anaesthetic. Direct the needle subcutaneously towards the supraorbital notch on one side and inject 5–7 ml of solution continuously as the needle is advanced 1 cm beyond the notch. Withdraw the needle and redirect towards the other supraorbital notch and repeat the injection.

Agent	Concn	Volume	Onset	Duration
Prilo	1%	5–7 ml	10 min	3–4 h
Bupiv	0.25%	5–7 ml	15 min	6–8 h

Head and neck

Supraorbital and supratrochlear nerve blocks

Injection at supraorbital foramen

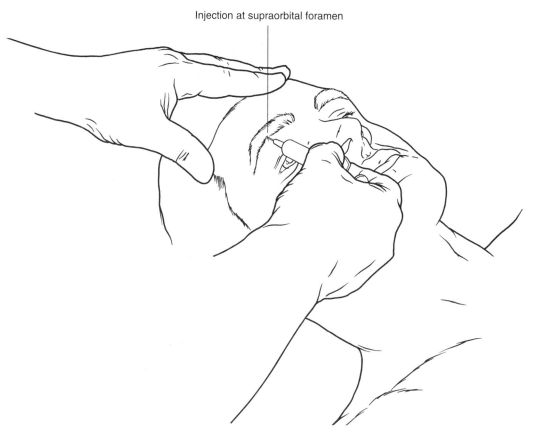

Fig. 3.53.1
Supraorbital nerve block

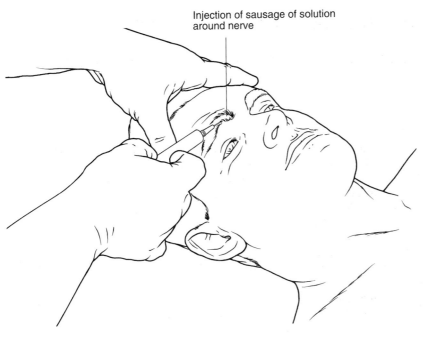

Injection of sausage of solution
around nerve

Fig. 3.53.2
Supratrochlear nerve block

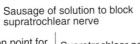

Sausage of solution to block
supratrochlear nerve

Needle insertion point for
supraorbital nerve block

Supratrochlear nerve

Supraorbital nerve

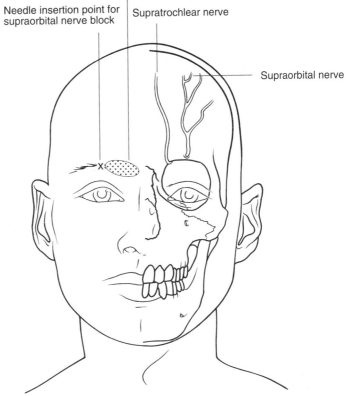

Fig. 3.53.3
Supraorbital and supratrochlear
nerve blocks, anterior view

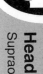

Topical anaesthesia

Landmarks
  Cornea
  Conjunctival reflection

Instruct the patient to look straight ahead and hold the eyelids open with the thumb and forefinger of one hand (Fig. 3.54.1). Drop one or two drops of local anaesthetic solution onto the cornea which will become anaesthetised almost instantly. Concentrated solutions cause marked stinging and the first drops can be made with diluted solution which is equally effective on the cornea. After 15–30 seconds, instil a few more drops concentrated solution into the conjunctival reflection, which may need several repeated instillations (a few drops at a time).

Agent	Concn	Volume	Onset	Duration
Ameth	1%	drops	rapid	15 min
Lido	2%	drops	rapid	15 min

Blockade for intraocular surgery

Retrobulbar or peribulbar?

The retrobulbar approach has been the mainstay of ophthalmic regional anaesthesia since it was first described by Knapp in 1884. It is, however, associated with a number of complications (Table 3.2) some of which are serious and can cause abandonment of the surgery, blindness and death. In an attempt to reduce the risk of serious complications, the peribulbar technique was described in 1986 as an alternative and possibly safer block and is becoming increasingly popular, especially with anaesthetists who perceive it as having a reduced risk of retrobulbar haemorrhage leading to abandonment of the procedure.

The retrobulbar approach requires only one injection, needs only a small volume of local anaesthetic, works within a few minutes and offers reliable motor and sensory blockade (Figure 3.55.1). It does require a supplementary facial nerve block and carries an appreciable risk of serious complications.

The peribulbar approach usually requires at least two intraocular injections (but not a separate facial nerve block), takes longer to work and requires larger volumes of local anaesthetic (Figure 3.55.2). It also carries with it the same risks as the retrobulbar approach but experience to date suggests that the incidence of serious complications is lower.

Table 3.2 Complications of ophthalmic regional anaesthesia

Complication	Cause
retrobulbar haemorrhage	intraconal vessel trauma
unconsciousness and cardiorespiratory collapse	intradural cuff injection vasovagal syncope local anaesthetic toxicity
blindness/optic atrophy	retinal vein/artery injection retrobulbar haemorrhage
retinal detachment	globe penetration
ocular muscle paresis	intramuscular injection drug toxicity

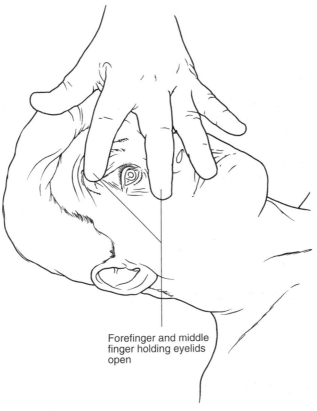

Forefinger and middle
finger holding eyelids
open

Fig. 3.54.1
Topical anaesthesia

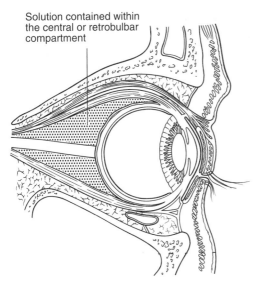

Solution contained within
the central or retrobulbar
compartment

Fig. 3.55.1
Retrobulbar block, cross section view (distribution of
solution)

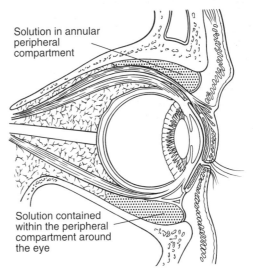

Solution in annular
peripheral
compartment

Solution contained
within the peripheral
compartment around
the eye

Fig 3.55.2
Peribulbar block, cross section view (distribution of
solution)

Retrobulbar block

Landmarks
- Sclerocorneal junction (limbus)
- Inferior conjunctival reflection

With the patient lying supine, anaesthetise the cornea and conjunctiva topically as described previously. Ask the patient to look straight ahead and then insert a 3.5 cm 25 G needle through the conjunctival reflection vertically below the lateral limbus (Fig. 3.56.1). Initially, direct the needle in a sagittal plane parallel to the floor of the orbit, with the bevel of the needle facing the globe, until the equator of the globe is passed (approximately 10–15 mm depth) and then redirect the needle slightly medially and upwards to enter the muscle cone, usually at a depth of 30 mm (Figs 3.56.2, 3.56.3). If the globe should deviate suddenly or the patient complains of ocular pain, the needle is in danger of penetrating the globe and should be carefully withdrawn immediately and then re-aligned. After careful aspiration inject 3 ml of solution slowly, withdraw the needle gradually and apply firm pressure with a pad for a few minutes before applying a gauze pad and a Honan's balloon inflated to 20 mmHg for 20 min. This disperses the local anaesthetic and lowers the intraorbital and intraocular pressures.

Some practitioners make the initial injection through the lower eyelid, in line with the lateral limbus. For this technique, an initial intradermal weal of local anaesthetic is required before making the same approach as outlined above. There are a variety of 'cocktails' used for retrobulbar block but the following mixture works well. Equal volumes of 2% lidocaine and 0.75% bupivacaine to a total of 5 ml to which some practitioners add 5 IU/ml hyaluronidase and some also add 5 µg/ml of adrenaline to improve drug distribution within the orbit and produce vasoconstriction unless it is contraindicated.

Agent	Concn	Volume	Onset	Duration
Bupiv and	0.75%	3–5 ml	5 min	6–12 h
Lido	2%			
See text for other combinations				

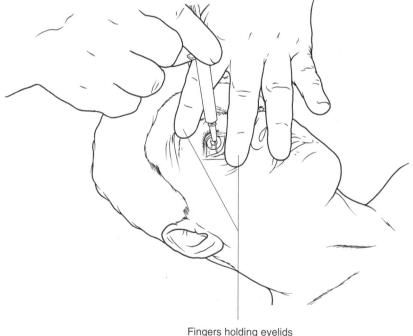

Fingers holding eyelids open

Fig. 3.56.1
Retrobulbar block

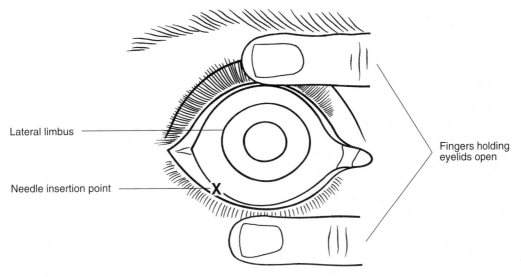

Fig. 3.56.2
Retrobulbar block, anterior view

Lateral limbus

Needle insertion point

X

Fingers holding
eyelids open

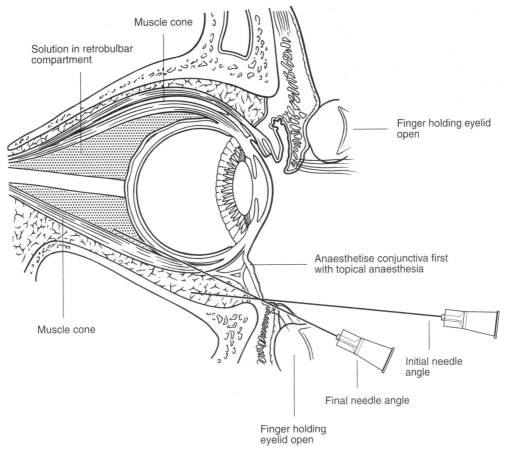

Muscle cone

Solution in retrobulbar
compartment

Finger holding eyelid
open

Anaesthetise conjunctiva first
with topical anaesthesia

Muscle cone

Initial needle
angle

Final needle angle

Finger holding
eyelid open

Fig. 3.56.3
Retrobulbar block, cross section view

Facial nerve block

This nerve block is often required to supplement a retrobulbar block but should not be necessary after peribulbar block. The large volume of local anaesthetic solution used in the peribulbar block results in penetration of the eyelids directly and therefore there is no need for a separate injection into the facial nerve branches.

Landmarks
Lateral margin of orbit

Insert a 25 G needle 1 cm lateral to the lateral margin of the orbit and raise an intradermal weal. From this point, slowly inject local anaesthetic solution down to the periosteum and then re-angle the needle towards the prominence of the cheekbone, slowly injecting 2–3 ml as the needle is advanced (Fig. 3.57.1). Withdraw the needle to the skin weal and direct it superiorly and slowly inject a further 2–3 ml of solution as the needle is advanced directly cephalad (Figs 3.57.2, 3.57.3). This blocks the temporal and zygomatic branches of the facial nerve and, by not injecting into the eyelids, the localised bleeding into the eyelids which can occur with other methods is avoided. The entire facial nerve can be blocked before it divides into its terminal branches at the level of the temporomandibular joint. This results in all the facial muscles being blocked which can distress patients and is unnecessary for eye surgery.

Agent	Concn	Volume	Onset	Duration
Bupiv + adren	0.5%	6 ml	15 min	6 h

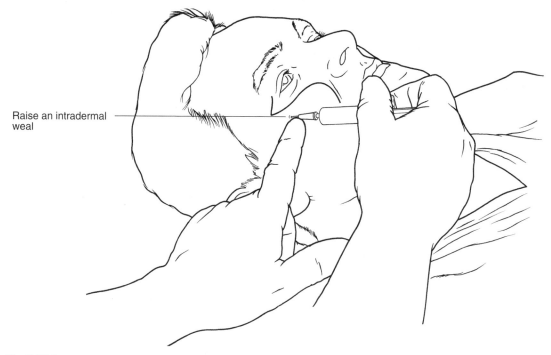

Raise an intradermal weal

Fig. 3.57.1
Facial nerve block

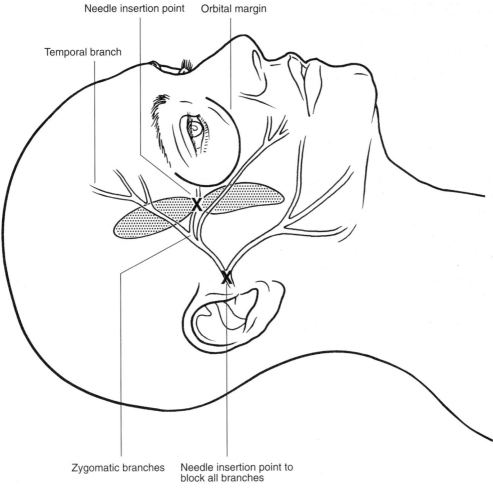

Temporal branch

Needle insertion point   Orbital margin

X

X

Zygomatic branches   Needle insertion point to
                       block all branches

Fig. 3.57.2
Facial nerve block, lateral view

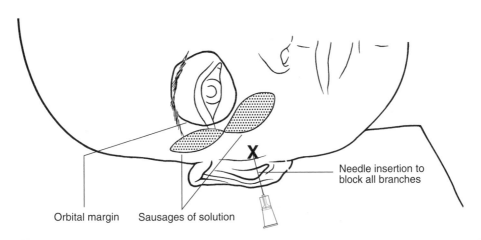

X

Needle insertion to
block all branches

Orbital margin   Sausages of solution

Fig. 3.57.3
Facial nerve block, anterior view

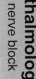

Peribulbar block

Landmarks
- Lateral corneoscleral junction
- Inferior conjunctival reflection
- Medial limbus
- Upper eyelid
- Inner canthus

Position the patient supine with their gaze fixed straight ahead. Anaesthetise the cornea and conjunctiva as described on pages 154–155 and then introduce a 25 G needle through the conjunctival reflection vertically below the lateral limbus, parallel to the floor of the orbit and tangential to the globe (Fig. 3.58.1). If the needle strikes bone, slightly redirect so that the tip of the needle is safely positioned outside the muscle cone, close to the orbital wall beyond the equator of the globe at a depth of about 2.5 cm. After careful aspiration, slowly inject 5 ml of chosen mixture and closely observe the globe and surrounding structures. If the conjunctiva swells quickly, the needle is too superficial and needs to be re-positioned (although there will be some enlargement of the conjunctiva and lower eyelid as the full volume is injected). Withdraw the needle slowly and apply light pressure to the eye with a soft pad (Fig. 3.58.2).

Only a minority of patients will have a complete motor and sensory block after a single injection. By testing individual muscle movements after 5 min, appropriate supplementary blocks can be administered to complete the technique

(Fig. 3.58.3). Most commonly, a second injection is made in the supero-nasal area by inserting the same needle through the upper eyelid vertically above the medial limbus to a depth of 2 cm aiming tangentially away from the globe (Fig. 3.58.4). Alternatively, the second injection may be made through the conjunctiva in the medial canthus, medial to the caruncle, the needle being inserted parallel to the medial wall of the orbit. Inject up to 5 ml of local anaesthetic solution after careful aspiration and then apply a pad and a Honan's balloon inflated to 20 mmHg for 20 min to disperse the local anaesthetic and reduce intraocular pressure.

As a consequence of the large volumes used, the local anaesthetic solution penetrates the eyelids directly and therefore there is no need for a separate injection into the facial nerve branches.

Agent	Concn	Volume	Onset	Duration
Bupiv and Lido	0.75% 2%	10 ml total	30 min	4–6 h

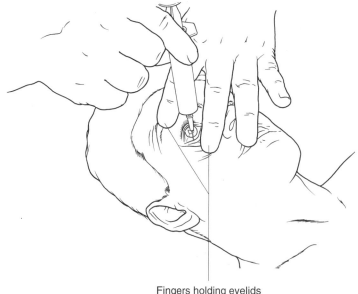

Fingers holding eyelids open

Fig. 3.58.1
Peribulbar block

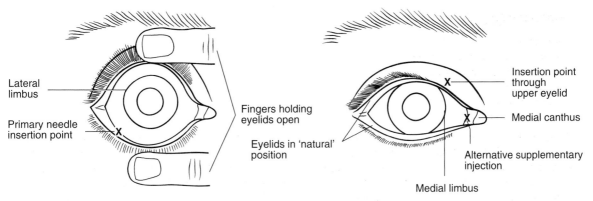

Fig. 3.58.2
Peribulbar block, anterior view (primary injection)

Fig. 3.58.3
Peribulbar block, anterior view (supplementary injections)

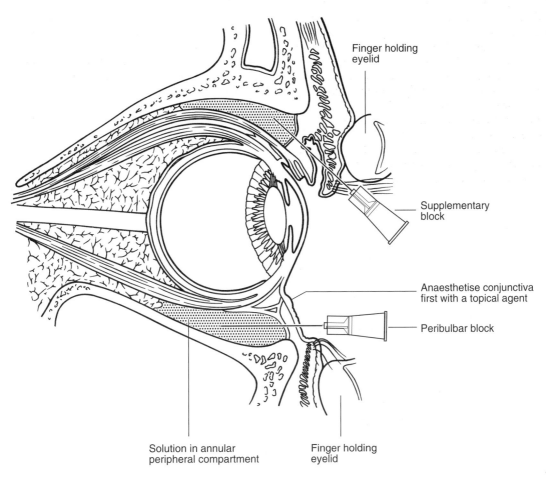

Fig. 3.58.4
Peribulbar block, cross section view

Continuous catheter techniques

Introduction

The duration of peripheral nerve blockade available from an isolated injection of local anaesthetic varies from 3 to 24 hours or more depending on the drug used, the concentration and volume of that drug and the nerve or plexus being blocked. This flexibility of duration is a major benefit of regional anaesthesia and for the majority of indications provides an adequate length of analgesia.

There are a number of clinical conditions where prolonged peripheral nerve block is advantageous and in these circumstances it is possible to offer several days or even weeks of peripheral nerve blockade by the use of catheter techniques whereby a fine gauge catheter is introduced into the sheath surrounding the nerve or plexus. This is similar to the use of continuous epidural catheter techniques. Suitable techniques for use with catheters are shown in Table 3.3.

Table 3.3 Continuous catheter techniques

Technique	Approach
brachial plexus	subclavian perivascular axillary
intercostal	unilateral single or multiple spaces
interpleural	interpleural
paravertebral	thoracic lumbar psoas compartment
femoral	femoral
sciatic	classical (Labat)

Benefits

Prolonged analgesia

There are few peripheral surgical conditions that require prolonged analgesia post-operatively. Patients undergoing major orthopaedic procedures such as total knee replacement or ligament reconstruction, may require continuous passive movement and physiotherapy for the first 24–48 hours. This treatment will be much better tolerated if the patient has a prolonged femoral nerve (and preferably sciatic) blockade. Brachial plexus catheter techniques may be used to provide prolonged analgesia after complex reconstruction of the forearm and hand. For post-operative management of major thoraco-lumbar surgery, intercostal, interpleural, paravertebral and lumbar plexus catheter techniques have been described. Chronic pain conditions, either due to malignancy, ischaemia or reflex sympathetic dystrophy can be more effectively managed once prolonged analgesia with peripheral nerve catheters has been achieved.

Sympathetic blockade

Brachial plexus, femoral and sciatic nerve blockade induce a widespread sympathectomy in the affected limb for the duration of the somatic sensory and motor block. Perfusion of the limb will improve, which may be important in the management of traumatised limbs undergoing reconstruction, by increasing the blood supply to areas of critical perfusion, for example skin flaps and end arteries. After major vascular surgery, evidence suggests that the incidence of graft failure is significantly reduced by regional anaesthesia. This is thought to be due to both improved blood flow to the graft and reduced reflex thrombogenic response following surgery. In patients with ischaemic rest pain of the lower limb, it is often possible to improve the blood supply to areas of critical perfusion so that in addition to alleviating the pain, any surgery that may be required can be planned more effectively.

Improved patient management

Effective peripheral nerve blockade will abolish the need for opioid drugs with concomitant benefits to patient management. Chronic pain conditions may be opioid resistant with the result that patients need high doses of opioids thus inducing many of the well recognised side effects, yet providing sub-optimal analgesia. If additional background analgesia is still required after an apparently successful regional technique, a combination of non-steroidal anti-inflammatory drugs (NSAIDs) and small doses of opioids will prove sufficient. For patients who have painful limbs with restricted movement, continuous analgesia techniques allow active rehabilitation and physiotherapy to restore limb and joint function. This has a profound benefit on the patient's psychological state as well as improving limb function.

Catheter techniques

Equipment

Cannula over needle

Parallel-sided intravenous cannulae (18 G) should be used for the axillary approach to the brachial plexus. If a peripheral nerve stimulator is used to locate the plexus, use a cannulated needle with a steel hub or alternatively, insert a fine gauge hypodermic needle into the proximal end of the needle shaft and use it as the contact for the stimulator. Take care when placing the cannula because the needle tip is designed to cut.

Epidural needle and catheter

Tuohy needles and epidural catheters may be used for the supraclavicular approaches to the brachial plexus, intercostal, interpleural, paravertebral, femoral and sciatic techniques. The needle is non-cutting and thus it is unlikely to result in nerve damage and will give tactile information during insertion. The main disadvantage is that the catheter is unstiffened and may not advance satisfactorily along the nerve sheaths.

Seldinger-type intravascular catheters

These may be used instead of epidural needles and have the advantages of making smaller holes with the introducing needle and wire. Having the catheter stiffened by the wire enables it to be directed with more accuracy. A 16 or 18 G 20 cm length catheter is especially suitable for femoral and sciatic nerve blockade.

Radiological confirmation

The introduction and final positioning of catheters can be facilitated by the use of an image intensifier and a suitable water soluble X-ray contrast medium.

Techniques

Standard approaches to most nerves are suitable for inserting catheters although minor modifications may be necessary. In the majority of cases, once the needle is correctly positioned, a 10 ml injection of normal saline is used to open up the perineural space and allow the catheter to be introduced more easily.

The procedure must be carried out under full sterile precautions to minimise the risk of introducing infection into the nerve sheath during the insertion and subsequently along the catheter track. Once the catheter or cannula is in place it must be secured (preferably with a suture) and covered with a transparent occlusive dressing.

Brachial plexus

For the subclavian perivascular approach, an epidural needle gives the most obvious sensation of resistance as it pierces the fascial sheath and the needle orifice is aligned so that the catheter is directed distally along the plexus. The plexus is normally less than 3 cm beneath the skin, so once the sheath is entered, carefully advance the catheter 2–3 cm into the plexus.

The axillary approach should be performed with an intravenous cannula. The needle is sharp and long bevelled and will not provide much resistance to advancement through the sheath. As soon as paraesthesiae are elicited or pulse synchronous muscle movements are stimulated, immobilise the needle and carefully advance the cannula sheath. A short extension tube can be attached before the cannula is secured to the skin.

Intercostal nerve

'Walk' an 18 G epidural needle off the caudal edge of the rib and advance it 3–4 mm into the space surrounding the neurovascular bundle. With the bevel facing medially, advance the catheter 3 cm towards the paravertebral space. There are reports of a failure rate of 20% with the catheters lying superficial to the space or within the pleural cavity, thus giving an interpleural block. Although a single catheter will block up to 5 dermatomes, the pattern of block is very variable and two catheters may be necessary for extensive surgery or trauma.

Interpleural block

A catheter technique is described on pages 104–105.

Paravertebral and psoas compartment blocks

Using the standard approaches described in Section 3, a 16 G Tuohy needle is used to locate the compartment and an epidural catheter is introduced 2–3 cm into the compartment.

Catheter techniques

Femoral nerve block

Use a 20 cm 16 G Seldinger needle kit in conjunction with a peripheral nerve stimulator so that the nerve can be accurately located without relying on paraesthesiae from the cutting needle bevel. Immobilise the needle and distend the nerve sheath with an injection of normal saline to allow easy advancement of the wire. The wire should pass easily up the femoral sheath and the catheter subsequently be advanced over the wire towards the lumbar plexus.

Sciatic nerve block

The classical approach of Labat is the easiest approach to use because the needle can be introduced more closely to the long axis of the nerve than other techniques which approach the nerve more distally and at right angles, allow. A Tuohy needle or a Seldinger kit can be used. Note that the technique can be difficult with either method. It is most important to distend the perineural space, having carefully located the nerve with a nerve stimulator. It may not be possible to introduce more than 2–3 cm of catheter but provided that it is securely fixed, this will be sufficient.

Injection and infusion volumes

The normal drug concentration and volumes can be used to establish the block. If rapid onset is required, use prilocaine 2% and then bupivacaine. Repeated bolus injections may be appropriate as sensation begins to return. Alternatively, a continuous infusion can be used to follow the initial injection absorption. The arguments for repeated injections or infusions are the same as those applied to epidural analgesia. Infusions provide more continuous analgesia with fewer interventions by the attending staff and may use a lower total dose in 24 hours, but the block may regress unless the infusion rate is carefully adjusted. The risk of systemic absorption is ever present and toxicity must be continually monitored, particularly if additional boluses are required.

The role of opioid drugs in peripheral nerve blockade is controversial. Fentanyl has been reported as being effective in sciatic and femoral nerve infusions and morphine has been added to intra-articular bupivacaine with resulting benefit for arthroscopic surgery.

Continuous Catheter techniques

Section 4

Reference

Abbreviations

ACTH   adrenocortico-trophic hormone

Adren   adrenaline

Ameth   amethocaine

ASIS   anterior superior iliac spine

Bupiv   bupivacaine

CN   cranial nerve

CNS   central nervous system

Concn   concentration

CPR   cardiopulmonary resuscitation

CSF   cerebro spinal fluid

CVS   cardiovascular system

EMIS   Education and Medical Illustration Services

EMLA   eutectic mixture of local anaesthetics

ENT   ear nose and throat

FRC   functional residual capacity

LCNT   lateral cutaneous nerve of the thigh

Lido   lidocaine

NSAID   non-steroidal anti-inflammatory drug

PEFR   peak expiratory flow rate

PNS   peripheral nerve stimulator

Prilo   prilocaine

Further reading

Principles and practice
Rational use of peripheral nerve blockade

Bach S, Noreng M F, Tjelldeu N U 1988 Phantom limb pain in amputees during the first twelve months following limb amputation after pre-operative lumbar epidural blockade. Pain 33: 297–301

Christopherson R, Beattie C H et al 1993 Peri-operative morbidity in patients randomised to epidural or general anesthesia for lower extremity vascular surgery. Anesthesiology 179: 422–434

Fischer H B J 1995 Acute pain relief – the role of regional anaesthesia. CACC 6(2): 87–91

McClure J H, Wildsmith J A W 1991 Conduction blockade for post-operative analgesia. Edward Arnold, London

Tuman K J, McCarthey R J et al 1991 Effects of epidural anesthesia and analgesia on coagulation and outcome after major vascular surgery. Anesth Analg 73: 696–704

Equipment

BS 5081 Part 2 1987 Sterile hypodermic needles for single use. BSI standards, Milton Keynes

Moore D C, Mulroy A F, Thompson G E 1994 Peripheral nerve damage and regional anaesthesia. Br J Anaesth 73(4): 435–436

Pither C E, Raj P P, Ford D J 1985 The use of peripheral nerve stimulators for regional anesthesia. A review of experimental characteristics, technique, and clinical applications. Regional Anesthesia 10: 49–58

Rice A S, McMahon S B 1992 Peripheral nerve injury caused by injection needles used in regional anaesthesia: influence of bevel configuration studied in a rat model. Br J Anaesth 69(5): 433–438

Selander D, Dhuner K G, Lundborg G 1977 Peripheral nerve injury due to injection needles used for regional anaesthesia. Acta Anaesth Scand 21: 182–188

Winnie A P 1969 An 'Immobile Needle' for nerve blocks. Anesthesiology 31: 577–578

Local anaesthetic drugs

ABPI Data Sheet Compendium 1995–1996 Datapharm Publications Ltd., London

British National Formulary number 30 1995 British Medical Association and Royal Pharmaceutical Society of Great Britain, London

Dundee J W, Clarke R S J, McCaughey W 1991 Clinical anaesthetic pharmacology. Churchill Livingstone, Edinburgh 283–293

Richards A, McConachie I 1995 The pharmacology of local anaesthetic drugs. CACC 6(1): 41–47

Operative site

Anderson J E 1978 Grant's atlas of anatomy 7th edn. The Williams & Wilkins Company, Baltimore

Last R J 1972 Anatomy regional and applied 5th edn. Churchill Livingstone, Edinburgh

Pansky B, House E L 1975 Review of gross anatomy 3rd edn. Macmillan Publishing Co. Inc., New York.

Williams P L, Warwick R, Dyson M, Bannister L H (eds) 1989 Gray's anatomy, 37th edn. Churchill Livingstone, Edinburgh.

Techniques
Foot and ankle

Brown D L 1992 Atlas of regional anaesthesia. W B Saunders Company, Philadelphia 115–120

Cousins M J, Bridenbaugh P O (eds) 1988 Neural blockade in clinical anaesthesia and management of pain 2nd edn. Lippincott, Philadelphia 434–437

Mulroy M F 1989 Regional anaesthesia. Little, Brown & Company, Boston 199–205

Scott D B 1989 Techniques of regional anaesthesia. Appleton & Lange, Norwalk 134–140

Lower limb

Brown D L 1992 Atlas of regional anaesthesia. W B Saunders Company, Philadelphia 73–114

Cousins M J, Bridenbaugh P O (eds) 1988 Neural blockade in clinical anaesthesia and management of pain 2nd edn. Lippincott, Philadelphia 417–434

Scott D B 1989 Techniques of regional anaesthesia. Appleton & Lange, Norwalk 116–134

Wildsmith J A, Armitage E N 1991 Principles and practice of regional anaesthesia. Churchill Livingstone, Edinburgh 189–199

Femoral nerve block – '3 in 1'

Winnie A P, Rammamurthy S, Durrani A 1973 The inguinal paravascular technic of lumbar plexus anaesthesia; the '3 in 1' block. Anesth. Analg 52: 989–996

Sciatic nerve block

Labat G 1924 Regional anesthesia: its technic and clinical applications. W B Saunders Company, Philadelphia

Lumbar plexus block – psoas compartment

Chayen D, Nathan H, Chayen M 1976 The psoas compartment block. Anesthesiol 45: 95–99

Abdomen and thorax

Brown D L 1992 Atlas of regional anaesthesia. W B Saunders Company, Philadelphia 201–225, 235–238

Cousins M J, Bridenbaugh P O (eds) 1988 Neural blockade in clinical anaesthesia and management of pain 2nd edn. Lippincott, Philadelphia 510–529

Scott D B 1989 Techniques of regional anaesthesia. Appleton & Lange, Norwalk 44–46, 134–154, 154–159

Interpleural block

Scott P V 1991 Interpleural regional anaesthesia: detection of the interpleural space by saline infusion. Br J Anaesth 66: 131–133

Upper limb

Cousins M J, Bridenbaugh P O (eds) 1988 Neural blockade in clinical anaesthesia and management of pain 2nd edn. Lippincott, Philadelphia 384–416

Mulroy M F 1989 Regional anaesthesia. Little, Brown & Company, Boston 151–171, 179–184

Wildsmith J A, Armitage E N 1991 Principles and practice of regional anaesthesia. Churchill Livingstone, Edinburgh 169–184

Brachial plexus block

Fischer H B J 1990 Brachial plexus anaesthesia. CACC 1(2): 128–132

Scott D B 1989 Techniques of regional anaesthesia. Appleton & Lange, Norwalk 90–110

Winnie A P 1983 Plexus anaesthesia Vol 1. Perivascular techniques of brachial plexus block. Schultz, Copenhagen

Suprascapular nerve block

Wasseff M R 1992 Suprascapular nerve block. A new approach for the management of frozen shoulder. Anaesthesia 47: 120–123

Hand and wrist

Brown D L 1992 Atlas of regional anaesthesia. W B Saunders Company, Philadelphia 52–54

Scott D B 1989 Techniques of regional anaesthesia. Appleton & Lange, Norwalk 112–114

Wildsmith J A, Armitage E N 1991 Principles and practice of regional anaesthesia. Churchill Livingstone, Edinburgh 183–184

Head and neck

Brown D L 1992 Atlas of regional anaesthesia. W B Saunders Company, Philadelphia 121–153

Cousins M J, Bridenbaugh P O (eds) 1988 Neural blockade in clinical anaesthesia and management of pain 2nd edn. Lippincott, Philadelphia 533–560

Scott D B 1989 Techniques of regional anaesthesia. Appleton & Lange, Norwalk 56–72

Wildsmith J A, Armitage E N 1991 Principles and practice of regional anaesthesia. Churchill Livingstone, Edinburgh 203–213

Ophthalmology

Brown D L 1992 Atlas of regional anaesthesia. W B Saunders Company, Philadelphia 157–164

Cousins M J, Bridenbaugh P O (eds) 1988 Neural blockade in clinical anaesthesia and management of pain 2nd edn. Lippincott, Philadelphia 577–592

Scott D B 1989 Techniques of regional anaesthesia. Appleton & Lange, Norwalk 78–86

Wildsmith J A, Armitage E N 1991 Principles and practice of regional anaesthesia. Churchill Livingstone, Edinburgh 213–221

Index of specific techniques

General index

---

usra.ca